PATHWAYS IN MEDICINE

PATHWAYS IN MEDICINE

A Journal of Topics in Medicine in the Spirit of Halacha and Jewish Thought

Translated and arranged by
Paltiel Roodyn
M.A. (Oxon), B.A. Hons. (London)

Laniado Hospital
Kiryat Sanz
Netanya, Israel

ISBN 1-56871-060-7

Phototypeset at Targum Press
Printing plates by Frank, Jerusalem

Trade distribution:
Feldheim Publishers
200 Airport Executive Park
Nanuet, N.Y. 10954

Trade distribution in Israel:
Targum Press Ltd.
POB 43170
Jerusalem 91430

Printed in Israel

Preface

Fourteen years ago, the International Friends of Sanz Medical Center Laniado Hospital undertook to finance the Hebrew publication of a journal devoted to topics on medicine in the spirit of Halachah and Jewish thought. The journal, known as *BeShvilei HaRefuah — Pathways in Medicine —* was extraordinarily well received by rabbis, doctors, scholars, and a large segment of our friends and supporters.

Through the gracious generosity of Mr. and Mrs. Ervin Landau of London, England, we are printing an English version of selected articles, which have appeared in previous issues.

It is our sincere hope that this volume will enhance the reader's interest in the Halachic aspects of medicine and provide insight into some typical problems and challenges which are encountered in medical institutions such as Sanz Medical Center Laniado Hospital.

Shevat 5755
Rabbi Meier S. Eisemann
International Friends of
S.M.C. Laniado Hospital
Netanya, Israel

Table of Contents

Translator's Preface

When I was asked to translate, edit and arrange excerpts from articles which had been published in the journal *Pathways in Medicine*, I little realised that I was about to enter upon a voyage of discovery which would prove to be as interesting as it was enjoyable. The great Rabbis who have contributed to this journal have given their rulings on many halachic problems concerning the day-to-day running of a modern hospital: Could a new form of digital thermometer be used on the Sabbath? What is the connection between psychiatry and the Torah? What are the rulings of the Torah about test-tube babies, donation of eggs to an infertile woman, or the problems of abortion or mercy killing? These problems in medical ethics are currently under discussion in the non-Jewish world, which is also seeking solutions to the moral and ethical issues involved.

With thanks to Hashem, we, the Jewish people, need have no hesitation or doubt as to how to approach ethical problems. The Torah gives us sure guidance, as we can see from the detailed and clear rulings of our great Rabbis, which appear in this journal.

Soon after I began my work, I realised that, owing to the limitations of space, it would only be possible to translate and arrange excerpts from the mass of material available. In addition, the Rabbis wrote halachic decisions in precise and concise Hebrew, so the task often became one of explanation and enlargement rather than translating word-for-word. I recalled the task of the Metargem, often mentioned in the Talmud. He would stand near a great Rabbi and expand and expound his words to the assembled students. The Rabbi himself would utter only short phrases. The task of the Metargem was to ensure that the audience understood the Rabbi's thoughts and ideas. I have, therefore, tried to present to the English reader an elucidation and explanation of the great Rabbi's writings as they appeared in the journal, rather than a word-for-word translation.

A word of warning: it is not possible to make actual halachic decisions concerning personal medical problems from this translation. In every case of doubt, a Rabbi should be asked! Personal or individual halachic decisions should not *be made on the basis of this translation.*

However, it is possible to obtain from this work an understanding of the lofty principles on which such halachic rulings are based in each and every case.

The World Is Built on Torah Righteousness

**HaRav Y. Halberstam, *ztz"l*,
Grand-Rabbi of Sanz-Klausenberg**

Excerpts from an address given by the Grand Rabbi of Sanz-Klausenberg, Rabbi Y. Halberstam, ztz"l, at the opening of the Second World Assembly of the Sanzer Hassidim and at the ceremony of the laying of the cornerstone of the new Medical Center at Kiryat Sanz, published in "Pathways in Medicine" 5 (Sivan 5741-June 1982).

Summary: The Admor of Klausenberg, *ztz"l*, relates how he made a promise that if Hashem would save him from the concentration camps in which he had been imprisoned, he would, on becoming free, found a hospital based on Torah principles of humanity and lovingkindness, in contrast to the wickedness which he had experienced. He gives thanks to Hashem that he was privileged to see his ambition realised.

My dear friends and honoured guests,

I give thanks to Hashem with a full heart that I have been privileged to come to our Holy Land and take part in this joyful religious ceremony — the laying of the cornerstone of the new Medical Center in Kiryat Sanz, twenty-five years after the foundation of Kiryat Sanz, with the help of the Almighty, blessed be His Name!

The duty to study the Torah is one of the commandments which relates to the relationship between man and his Creator, while the duty to be merciful refers to the lovingkindness that men show to their fellowmen. It is stated in the Book of Michah (6:8): "What the Lord requires of you is only to do justly and to love mercy." The Radak explains this verse by saying: "Loving mercy — this means showing an abundance of kindness towards one's fellowmen." In fact, Torah and lovingkindness are bound together by unbreakable bonds. Our Rabbis stated in the Mishnah (*Pirkei Avos* 3:21): "Without Torah there is no good behaviour, and where there is no good behaviour there is no Torah." It also states in Tractate *Derech Eretz* (8): "The only good behaviour is that shown by the wise," meaning that only a person who has acquired the wisdom of the Torah can truly be said to have acquired the secret of good behaviour. (See also *Kalah Rabati*, chap. 1).

Disbelief in Hashem was the inheritance of the non-Jewish, heretical nations of the world. Thus, when Cain killed his brother, Abel, he cried: "There is no Judge and there is no justice!" (See *Targum Yonatan Ben Uziel* on Bereshis 4:8.) This disbelief in Hashem was the direct cause of the terrible deterioration in humanity that finally led to the murder of a brother. Without fear of Hashem, there is no holding back; there is no brake on the bodily desires of a human being. As it says in the Book of Job (11:12), "A man is born like a wild ass." Our forefather Avraham also said (Bereshis 20:11): "I said surely the fear of God is not in this place, and they will slay me for my wife's sake!"

It is clear to anyone with understanding that if there is no faith in Hashem, the Ruler of the world, Who knows the most secret and the most hidden thoughts of every living creature, there is no foundation in humanity for "good manners," or so called "good relationships" between human beings. The reason is that the "gentlemanly" ways which disbelievers invent do not stand up to difficulty or opposition! As soon as "good manners" come into conflict with their desires or preferences, or interfere with their comfort, they discard "idealism" and abandon "good relationships."

We felt this personally when we suffered under the rule of that accursed power, the German Nazis, may their name be blotted out! With our own eyes we witnessed what took place during those years of terrible bloodshed in Europe — a Europe which called itself "enlightened" and "advanced," where everyone was "civilised" and "cultured." It was in just these countries that the most shameful degradation of humanity occurred! Their people were transformed into cruel, predatory beasts. Their cruelty was worse than anything that had been seen in the entire existence of the world.

Can we not see today before our very eyes what happened to the "movements" — communism, fascism and others — and where they led their followers? They proudly stood up and waved their flags in honour of such slogans as the "brotherhood of man," "peace forever" and "social equality." In a short time, they turned into forces of destruction, dragging down humanity. The whole world was caught up in an unparalleled wave of depraved persecution the likes of which have never been seen before. It degraded the human spirit and destroyed the freedom of man. It was accompanied by an aggressive and violent conquest of whole nations throughout the world!

The Torah (Devarim 12:31) states, with reference to idol-worshippers: "Also their sons and their daughters do they burn in the fire to their gods." Rashi, citing the *Sifri*, says that "the word *also* comes to tell us that they do this *also* to their fathers and mothers. Rabbi Akiva said: 'I once saw a non-Jew pushing his own father in front of a dog, who began to eat him.' " No doubt, this action of the non-Jew, who was prepared to feed his hungry dog with the flesh of his own father, was motivated by feelings of "pure humanity" towards his beloved pet, who was suffering pangs of hunger; this touched his heart and troubled him, and it was more important to him than the life of his own father...

The three pillars on which the universe stands — learning of the Torah, observance of its commandments and performing lovingkindness to others — are in fact one unified concept

This was the way of life of our forefathers, the holy Rabbis, the pupils of the Baal Shem Tov, of blessed memory, who was known as the Light of Israel. They joined together in perfect harmony the study of the Torah, the observance of its commandments, and the performance of lovingkindness to their fellowmen. These are the *three* pillars on which the world stands. They are the foundations of the Universe. My late revered grandfather, the Admor of Sanz, the author of *Divrei Chayim*, was an outstanding example of a person who led this holy way of life.

Today, however, due to our many sins, the three pillars of the universe have become weak, and the words of Iyov (9:6) are being fulfiled: "He shakes the earth out of its place, and its pillars tremble." The Almighty is shaking the earth out of its foundations because the three pillars supporting the world have become weak. When these three pillars no longer stand as one, all the ways of the world become confused. Humanity becomes twisted, and the whole order of the world is overturned. These words refer to the way man behaves towards his fellowman — where a man, as it were, swallows his neighbour alive — as well as to relationships between the nations, who fight with each other and tear each other to pieces.

I saw with my own eyes the sufferings of our poor people beneath the rod of His anger. I suffered with my people in those camps, which were hell on earth, from the persecutions of that aggressive wicked power, the accursed Germans, may their name be blotted out! We were prisoners under their sword. With our own eyes we saw the depraved and evil actions of these "men of culture," actions which they planned down to the last detail, with their "scientific methods!" Then we could clearly see the difference between our kind of lovingkindness, based on the foundations of our Holy Torah, and the so-called kindness of the non-Jew: "When the non-Jew shows kindness, it is sin!" At that time I promised that if Hashem helped me and delivered me from that lion's den, from the shadow of death and evil, I would strive, with the help of the Almighty, to restore our days as of old and devote myself to holy deeds, emulating our forefathers: performing righteousness and justice, and holding to the ways of Hashem, the Tree of Life, striving to place on firm foundations those three pillars on which the world stands.

I must give thanks and praise to the Almighty that I was saved from that fearful Holocaust and that those dry bones came once more to life, the weak hands became strong, the bent knees were straightened, and I was one of that small remnant saved from the sea of blood. We were brands pulled from the flames! I was saved from His day of anger by His great kindness and succeeded in founding, with help from Heaven, "The Holocaust Survivors." This organisation was active in Germany,

Austria and France, and through the great kindness of Hashem, first in the transit camps, and later in the United States, succeeded in setting up Torah institutions and assisting thousands of families loyal to Hashem, to His Torah and to His people, who would strive to perpetuate the three pillars from generation to generation.

It is now twenty-five years since Hashem, in His goodness, accorded me the privilege of founding, in the land of our forefathers, our religious settlement of Jewish people faithful to Hashem and to His Torah. It was named after my late holy grandfather, the Rabbi and light of Israel, the Admor of Sanz, may his memory be a blessing. One of the most outstanding and famous institutions we founded is the Kiryat Sanz Hospital, which has worked, with the help of the Almighty, for a number of years, to bring help and succour and comfort and healing to every sick person who enters its gates. It strives to cure the sick out of love and humanity, in accordance with the commandment of the Almighty: "Thou shalt love thy neighbour as thou lovest thyself."

This hospital has shown itself capable of sanctifying the Name of Heaven in the eyes of the world. Its medical staff demonstrates that it is possible to provide the most up-to-date scientific medical treatment and *at the same time* scrupulously observe the Law of the Torah and the decisions of the Rabbis in every detail. So the Almighty promised us in His Torah (Shemos 15:26): "And He said: If you will diligently hearken to the voice of the Lord your God, and will do what is right in His eyes, and will give ear to His commandments, and *keep all His statutes*, all the diseases which I have put upon the Egyptians I will not place upon you, *for I am the Lord that healeth thee.*"

Today is the memorial day in honour of the crown of our

family, my father and teacher, the Admor of Rudnick, of blessed memory, who performed loving deeds for all Israel with all his heart and soul. He followed the example of Aharon the High Priest, who loved peace, pursued peace, loved his fellow-men and brought them near to Torah. He devoted all his life and strength to working for the good of the community and for the good of each individual in it. Here I wish to recall that only two weeks before he passed from this world, he wrote the following words to me: "Believe me, my dear son, when I say that I have never said a bad thing about any person." Is it not a wonderful thing to hear that a person could make such a statement about himself just before he passed away!

I give praise and thanks to the Creator of the Universe for all that has happened in the past, and for the fact that He granted me the privilege of being among the founders of this outstanding institution, which performs deeds of mercy and kindness for the individual and the community. My eyes are raised in prayer towards the Almighty, to pray for His help in the future and beg Him to grant us the privilege of strengthening our activities even more, in honour of his Blessed Name. I pray to Hashem, who has performed such kindness to me, that He send us His holy help so we may speedily complete this building, for the good of all Israel, and fulfil the words of Malachi (3:20): "But unto you that fear My name shall the sun of righteousness arise with healing in its wings." May Israel be saved by Hashem in everlasting salvation! Amen, and may this be His will!

The Torah of Lovingkindness

HaRav Y. Halberstam, *ztz"l*,
Grand Rabbi of Sanz-Klausenberg

Two years after Laniado Hospital, Kiryat Sanz, was opened, the medical staff visited the Grand Rabbi of Sanz-Klausenberg, Rabbi Y. Halberstam, ztz"l, in order to receive his blessing for their new work. Below are excerpts from the address which the Grand Rabbi gave to the staff. It was published in "Pathways in Medicine" 1 (Adar 5739 — March 1979).

Summary: The Grand Rabbi of Sanz-Klausenberg, *ztz"l*, blessed all the staff of the Hospital. He explained that just as the Torah is full of lovingkindness, so should a hospital also be filled with lovingkindness. Then it will be a Torah-true hospital, like Laniado, which is a true Torah institution.

The two tablets of stone on which the Ten Commandments were engraved are described in the Book of Devarim, chapter 10. The word for "tablets" in the Hebrew text is written in a slightly abbreviated form (the Hebrew letter *vav* is missing). Our Rabbis tell us, in the *Midrash Rabbah*, that this abbreviated form is in order to teach us that the two tablets were in fact designed to be thought of as one unified Tablet. The commandments associated with the relationship between a human being and his Creator — for example the prohibition against worshipping false gods and the commandment to honour the Sabbath — were engraved on the first tablet. On the second tablet were engraved laws associated with the relationship between man and his fellowmen — for example, the prohibitions against murder and theft. We learn from this that the laws dealing with the relationship between man and his fellowmen have the same status as the laws dealing with the relationship between man and his Creator. For example, the law prohibiting stealing has the same stringency and importance as the law forbidding the uttering of a false oath. If a Jewish employer wishes to know how to treat his employee, he has no need to turn to non-Jewish political philosophies and ideologies, like socialism or communism, for which so many people have given their lives. He can learn how men should treat their fellow human beings from the commandments of the Holy Torah, which teach us to love our neighbor and respect his human rights and which give us laws such as the prohibition against stealing, the strict injunction not to delay the payment of an employee's wage, to love all Israel, and many others.

In former days, when slavery was accepted throughout the world, the non-Jewish slave was treated harshly, far worse than black workers are treated in certain countries today. In ancient times, a slave was forced to work in chains indefinitely. In contrast, our Holy Torah tells us that a Hebrew slave could only work for a maximum of six years; he had to be freed in the seventh year. When he was freed, his master was compelled to send him away with money and with gifts. The Babylonian Talmud (*Kiddushin* 20) even states that "he who purchases a Hebrew slave, purchases a master to rule over him." For example, if the master possesses only one mattress, the Torah commands him to give it to his slave. The Torah states that the Hebrew slave must be given precedence over his master in all matters concerning living conditions and personal comfort.

The commandments which relate to healing of the sick and

relieving their suffering are some of the most important of all the commandments of our Holy Torah; they include, the commandments to heal the sick, to visit the sick, to love one's fellowman, and to do kindness to others. The person who carries out these commandments will receive his reward in this world, and, in addition, his reward will be renewed for him after his death and continue to be paid to him in far, far greater measure in the World to Come. The Torah relates that during the period of the exile in Egypt, the two Jewish midwives, Shifrah and Puah, were in fact Yocheved and Miriam, the greatest ladies of the generation. They served as midwives during one of the darkest epochs in the history of our people, and the whole section of the Torah which is devoted to them tells us of the great reward they received for their actions.

We thus see the enormous importance the Torah attaches to healing the sick and relieving their suffering. Throughout our history, some of the greatest leaders of our people have also been doctors. They include many of the great Rabbis quoted in the Talmud, the Rambam, the Ramban, Rabbenu Yonah and many, many others. These great men did not study medicine in order to acquire a profession. They practised with the sole aim of healing and relieving the sick.

I wish to reveal to you now that my immigration to the Land of Israel was fraught with many difficulties. I was ill, and my doctors advised me not to travel. However, because of my great love for the Land of Israel, and especially for Kiryat Sanz, I undertook the journey without my doctor's consent. I did write to my doctor, to explain to him that in this particular instance I felt compelled not to take his advice. I told him that I trusted that, in spite of his expert knowledge in the field of heart disease, he had not taken fully into account the healing power possessed by the Land of Israel. I explained that I, as a believing Jew, had complete faith in the Holy One, Blessed be He, and the Holiness of the Land of Israel. Therefore, because I thought that my journey was important for the good of our holy institutions in the Land of Israel, I came, and I have been able, in spite of my state of health, to work on behalf of our hospital and our community in the Holy Land.

When we establish a hospital, we try to ensure that it will be run with full and detailed observance of the laws of the Sabbath and the highest possible standards of kashrus, and that the medical staff and specialists employed in the hospital will be outstanding experts in their particular fields. In addition, we have another aim, which to me is the most vital one of all: all those who work in the hospital should be possessed of a warm Jewish heart! They should love the patient, and their aim should be to cure the *patient*, not merely to cure the *disease*! They should not think of improving their medical skills at the expense of the patient's suffering. To our sorrow, nowadays we see doctors who concentrate on curing the disease and do not care very much if the patient himself lives or dies.

In our hospital, the staff must treat their patients with the love they have for all Israel, and the love for one's neighbour, who was made in the image of his Creator. The doctor should rejoice when he succeeds in curing a patient, for he has relieved the patient's suffering and the suffering of the patient's family. The midwife should rejoice when she helps bring a living and healthy infant into the world. Every midwife should wish *"Mazel tov!"* to *herself* after every successful birth; she should feel as if the newborn infant were her own child!

All that I have said above is the foundation of this hospital. I have been asked many times to explain what the connection is between a rabbi and a hospital. It is clear that this hospital is a holy Torah institution. Our Torah is a Torah of lovingkindness. Everyone can understand that a rabbi, and indeed every believing Jew, wishes to establish Torah institutions. Everyone should therefore be able to understand why a rabbi established this hospital, which is, in fact a magnificent Torah institution.

Today, it gives me great satisfaction to know that this hospital has been functioning for two years. I give thanks to Hashem for His goodness to us all and for the fact that He has helped us to build up the hospital. I trust in Hashem that He will help us extend this hospital and build the new wards and departments which are already being planned. I pray that Hashem will help us build a department dedicated to the Angel Gabriel, who should stand at the side of every one of the medical staff and every patient, in order to hasten their recovery.

I wish to take this opportunity to mention that I have already received many reports, informing me to my great joy that the staff of the hospital, medical and administrative, all work with faith, devotion and hearts open to all who enter the Hospital. With gratitude to Hashem, I can now say that the fame of this Hospital has spread far and wide; this is because our staff have shown such warm feelings to the patients and their families. Hundreds of people who were treated in this Hospital felt impelled to come to me to tell me how well they were treated. We trust and pray that this positive approach will continue to develop more and more in the future.

I bless all the staff of this hospital and all who work for the hospital. May Hashem grant us the privilege of seeing the opening of many more wards and departments, and may Hashem bless you all with peace of mind, happiness and long life. Amen.

Principles of Administration of the Hospital

HaRav Y. Halberstam, *ztz"l,*
Grand Rabbi of Sanz-Klausenberg

These Principles of Administration were reprinted in "Pathways in Medicine" 1 (Elul 5739 - September 1979).

Summary: The Grand Rabbi of Sanz-Klausenberg, *ztz"l,* followed the procedure adopted by Rabbi Akiva Eger, of blessed memory, who founded a hospital in Posen in the year 1830. At that time, Rabbi Akiva Eger laid down seven or eight principles on which the administration of the hospital in Posen should be based. In spite of many difficulties and troubles, these principles remained the foundation of the hospital in Posen right up to the destruction of the Jewish communities there by the Germans in the Holocaust.

1. The Kiryat Sanz Hospital shall be established as a holy institution with the aim of bringing benefit and healing to those who suffer, in accordance with the commandments of the Torah as stated in Tractate *Nedarim* 41, and in the *Shulchan Aruch, Yoreh De'ah* 336.

2. The Hospital shall accept every patient without distinction of sex, religion or race.

3. The Hospital shall be established on the basis of complete faith in the Creator of the Universe, Who grants life to every

living creature, and in Whose hand is every living soul. Its doctors and medical staff shall have a firmly based faith in this basic principle, and all their practices shall be in accordance with a spirit of faith in the Creator and in His Holy Torah.

4. In this Hospital all the commandments of the Torah shall be observed, as laid down by the *Shulchan Aruch* and by our great Rabbis. A Rav learned in Torah shall be appointed, to whom all questions shall be put concerning religious practice, and his decisions shall be final and binding upon all the Hospital staff. In the matter of the observance of the Sabbath, the permission granted in the Torah to instruct non-Jews to carry out certain classes of work under certain conditions shall be made use of. Care shall be taken that the clothing worn by persons in the hospital shall be modest in accordance with the traditions of the Torah and Judaism.

5. Every effort shall be made to employ doctors and medical staff who are highly qualified in their profession, and who also possess good qualities in their mode of behaviour and in their attitude to life. They should be persons who are full of love for their fellow Jews and for every other human being. As it is stated in the Torah: "Thou shalt love thy neighbour as thyself."

6. All staff shall endeavour in every possible way to lessen the pain and suffering of the patients and seek to improve their inner feelings and spiritual condition, as this will also assist in their healing, as the *Shulchan Aruch* states.

7. Every effort shall be made to be very particular in the observance of the commandments relating to the treatment of one's fellowman, with special care not to do any wrong to any person who works in the Hospital, or comes into contact with the Hospital, and to be especially careful that all wages are paid at the correct time, without any delay.

8. The atmosphere in the hospital among the staff, and in their dealings with all whom they come into contact, shall be based on friendship, peace and brotherly love.

9. A Torah research institute shall be established to carry out research on solutions to medical problems in the light of the rulings of the Torah, in order to assist Jewish people who observe the commandments of the Torah.

The Practice of Medicine Fulfils Hashem's Wishes

HaRav Eliyohu Shmuel Schmerler,
Rosh Yeshiva, Sanz Yeshiva

Excerpts from an article in "Pathways in Medicine" 2 (Elul 5739 - September 1979).

Summary: Rabbi Schmerler analyses the religious principles on which Laniado Hospital is based.

First, I wish to quote from a letter written by the Admor, the Grand Rabbi of Sanz-Klausenberg, *ztz"l*, in which he states: "Human perfection cannot be acquired merely through human interrelations and etiquette, but only through obedience to the Will of Hashem. It is stated in Bereshis 18:19 that Hashem said of Abraham: 'He shall command his children and his household after him, that they may keep the way of Hashem to do righteousness and justice.' From this we learn that righteousness and justice are acquired only through following the way of Hashem, not merely from polite human behaviour."

It seems to me that these words are the spiritual foundation upon which Laniado Hospital in Kiryat Sanz is based. The purpose of this great work, which was made possible by the extreme devotion and self-sacrifice of the Admor, the Grand Rabbi of Sanz, *ztz"l*, was not merely to establish an institution in which the laws of the Sabbath and kashrus would be observed. It was based on the highest principles of lovingkindness exemplified by our Jewish heritage.

In the first chapter of *Pirkei Avos* we read: "The world rests upon three pillars: Torah, service and lovingkindness." True piety, or *chassidus*, is similarly based upon these three pillars: love of Hashem, love of His Torah, and love for the people of Israel.

At first sight it might appear that there is a distinction between the first two pillars — love of Hashem and His Torah, and the third pillar — love for the people of Israel. But from the Jewish point of view, there is no such distinction. According to the teachings of Sanz *chassidus*, the three pillars are bound together as one. The pillar of Torah is the basis of all three. Lovingkindness and love for the people of Israel is bound up with the ideals of Torah and service. Lovingkindness and love for the people of Israel is part of one's love for Hashem.

True kindness is based on complete obedience to the Will of Hashem. Kindness based only on human social rules is not on the same level. Thus the Talmud tells us: "The kindness of the nations is sin."

The Rambam states in the eighth chapter of *Hilchos Melachim* that the "seven laws given to the children of Noah" are in fact laws which can easily be understood by human intelligence, such as the prohibitions against stealing and murder. However, he adds, a righteous non-Jew "must obey them because they are the commandments of Hashem as handed down to Moshe. If he obeys them merely because his intelligence advises him to do so, he cannot be classed as being one of the wise and righteous among the nations."

The reason is that if such a person refrains from killing only because his intelligence tells him it is not right to kill, the next step will be "mercy killing." He will regard it as an ideal solution to certain problems. Then he will come to consider the killing of a baby in the womb a humanitarian act. The next step is to regard "genocide," in certain situations, as a benefit to humanity! True righteousness and justice can only be based on *complete* obedience to the laws of Hashem.

True love for the people of Israel derives its strength from love of Hashem and love of His Torah. These three principles are inseparably united, and each draws strength from the other.

This is the basis on which the Admor, the Grand Rabbi of Sanz-Klausenberg, *ztz"l*, founded the Laniado Hospital; to be an example of true lovingkindness in the world.

I recall the ceremony of laying the cornerstone of Laniado Hospital, when a visitor asked the Admor why he had decided to build the hospital on a site adjacent to the Kiryat Sanz Yeshiva. He replied that a law in the *Shulchan Aruch* states that a person who has a sick relative at home should visit the leading Rabbi in his town and ask him to pray to Hashem for mercy and for the recovery of the sick person. This law is found in the *Shulchan Aruch* before the laws relating to the practice of medicine by the doctor. From this we may learn that a hospital derives its spiritual strength and power to heal from the Torah, which emanates from the Yeshiva.

A hospital based on the principles elaborated in this article, with a great Torah scholar and Rabbi at its head, is bound to be successful in its fight against sickness and suffering. Similarly, the author of *Tosephos Yom Tov* founded a hospital in Prague, as did the great Rabbi Akiva Eger, who founded his own hospital in Posen. The fact that this hospital is ruled by the spirit of the righteous Rabbis and scholars of Torah will ensure that mere "rational" considerations will not be allowed to cause it to deviate from its path — true lovingkindness and following the wishes of Hashem.

This hospital is based on the principle that the doctor is a servant of Hashem. In his address, the Admor, the Grand Rabbi of Sanz, *ztz"l,* told the staff of the hospital: "Service in healing the sick — this is the path the doctors have chosen as a way of serving Hashem. This should be the aim of every doctor, pharmacist and nurse. Hashem, Who heals all flesh, Who has wrought miracles in order to heal the sick, has placed the power of healing in the hands of the doctors and of all those who work in the medical services. They are thus acting as agents of Hashem."

Washing a Patient with Hot Water on the Sabbath

HaRav Y. Halberstam, *ztz"l,*
Grand Rabbi of Sanz-Klausenberg

Excerpts from an article in "Pathways in Medicine" 5 (Sivan 5742 - June 1982).

Summary: The Grand Rabbi of Sanz-Klausenberg, *ztz"l*, concludes that it is permissible to use hot water to wash a patient who is suffering on the Sabbath, even though that patient's life is not in serious danger, provided, of course, that the water has been heated prior to the Sabbath and kept hot strictly according to the laws of Sabbath.

Question

Is it permissible to use hot water on the Sabbath to wash a patient who is suffering, but whose life is not in any way in danger?

Answer

Rabbi Akiva Eger, of blessed memory, stated that in his opinion it is permissible to use hot water to wash a patient who is suffering on the Sabbath. He notes that the *Shulchan Aruch* permits a non-Jew to carry water on the Sabbath through a courtyard where there is no *eruv* in order to wash a Jewish patient who is suffering. There is a discussion on this point among the Rabbis. Nearly all the Rabbis are of the opinion that the prohibition against washing with hot water on the Sabbath does not apply to the Festivals. From this we may, perhaps, learn that if a patient is suffering, it may even be permissible to wash him with hot water on the Sabbath. We learn that the reason for the prohibition against washing with hot water on the Sabbath was the risk that the bath attendant would forget and actually heat water on Sabbath for the patient. That is why this decree only applies to the Sabbath and not to a Festival, when water can be heated. If, then, the prohibition against washing with hot water on the Sabbath is more lenient than other prohibitions (which can only be broken for the sake of a patient whose life is in actual danger), it may well be that it is permissible to wash a patient who is only suffering, but is not dangerously ill, with hot water on the Sabbath.

In Tractate *Shabbos* 40, the case of a person suffering from a pain in the stomach is discussed. Some Rabbis say that in such a situation it is forbidden to place a glass bottle filled with hot water upon the person's stomach because the bottle filled with hot water might break, which would be like washing the sick person with hot water on the Sabbath. From this we might infer that it is forbidden to wash a patient's body with hot water on the Sabbath. On the other hand, one could say it *is*, in fact, permitted to wash a sick person who is suffering with hot water on the Sabbath, because, in the case of the glass bottle, if the hot water bottle broke it would not give comfort or help to the patient, whereas washing his body would help him. It may, therefore, be permissible to wash the patient with hot water on the Sabbath, even though the use of a glass hot water bottle, according to some Rabbis, is not.

Other cases where normally forbidden actions are permitted on the Sabbath in order to avoid suffering

There are other examples of actions which are usually forbidden on the Sabbath but permitted when human suffering would be caused. Thus, there is a prohibition against hunting or killing a living creature on Sabbath, but the *Shulchan Aruch* states that it is permissible to capture a flea on the body of a person because the person could suffer if it was not captured. The reason for this is that where a prohibition is not an extremely strict one, but has only been decreed to avoid a more serious infraction of the laws of Sabbath, then, in cases of suffering, the action could be permitted. We may conclude from this that because the prohibition against washing with hot water is not an extremely strict one, in cases where human suffering is involved, washing would be permissible.

Some Rabbis say that it is forbidden to untie a double knot on the Sabbath: a double knot may be regarded as "professionally tied," and such a knot must not be untied on the Sabbath. But the Rabbis do state that if leaving the knot tied on Sabbath would cause human suffering, it is permitted to untie it. One of the reasons for this conclusion is that it is not certain that a double knot is, in fact, a "professionally tied knot," the untying of which the Torah prohibits. Moreover, there are Rabbis who believe that *any* knot which was not *intended* to be permanent when it was tied may be untied on the Sabbath. Since the prohibition on untying such a knot is not a very strict one, where human suffering is involved, the Rabbis would permit untying the knot. The case of using hot water to wash a patient who is suffering on the Sabbath is similar.

Conclusion

We note that there are many cases where even a stricter Rabbinical prohibition (*shevus*) is not enforced by the Rabbis when human suffering is involved. We have seen that the prohibition against washing with hot water on the Sabbath is in a more lenient class of prohibitions. We must, therefore conclude that we should follow the ruling of Rabbi Akiva Eger quoted at the beginning of this discussion: the washing of a patient who is suffering may be carried out with hot water, even on the Sabbath, provided, of course, that the water has been heated before the Sabbath and kept hot strictly according to the laws of Sabbath.

The Jewish Meaning of Life

HaRav Asher Weiss,
Rosh Yeshiva, Sadegura, Bnei Brak

Extracts from an article in "Pathways in Medicine" 8 (Kislev 5747-January 1987).

Summary: Rabbi Weiss concludes that the true essence of life from the Jewish point of view is in the observance and study of the commandments of the Torah. He also emphasises the sanctity of life, which must be always uppermost in the minds of all staff serving in a religious hospital.

In chapter 18 of VaYikra we read: "You shall therefore keep My statutes and My ordinances, which if a man do, he shall live by them." This verse teaches us the meaning of the sanctity of life. On this verse, the Talmud (*Yoma* 85) comments: "The obligation to save a life overrules every other commandment of the Torah, since the verse states 'and he shall live by them,' and not die as a result of them."

The Rambam also comments on this verse in chapter 2 of *Hilchos Shabbos*: "From this we learn that the statutes of the Torah are not a form of retribution to the world, but are statutes of mercy, love and peace. To refute disbelievers who say that it is forbidden to violate the Sabbath in order to save a life, the Torah asks: 'Is it possible that I have given you laws that are not good, or statutes which will not preserve your lives?' "

The Talmud goes on to explain that one is permitted to

violate the laws of the Torah even in order to save the life of a terminally ill patient, who can only be expected to live a very short time.

Can we understand the secret of life?

The answer to this question is "No!" We can *never* understand the secret of life! The Torah states: "In truth, You are their Creator, and only You know the secret of their creation." Only the Creator, Who has given life to every living creature, knows the secret of life. In Bereshis (7:2) we read: "He breathed into his nostrils the breath of life." The *Zohar* explains this verse by saying, "the Creator breathed a part of Himself into man." The soul of a man is a part of Divinity. A man's soul comes from beneath the Throne of Glory of the Creator. We cannot understand the true essence of Divinity. The Torah tells us that Hashem stated, "And you shall not look upon Me and still live." Similarly, we cannot understand the true essence of the soul of a human being.

Just as we cannot understand the true nature of the human soul, we cannot understand how the soul, which is spiritual, can be joined to the body, which is material.

The Torah tells us that the souls of all the generations which were to be born were created on the first day of the Creation of the world. Rashi enlarges on this concept in his commentary on *Yevamos* 63: "In Heaven, there is a partition which divides the Creator from the Angels. Here are placed all the spirits and souls which were created during the Six Days of Creation." The soul of a human being was not created at the same time as his body; it is a separate creation. In *Sanhedrin* 91, the Talmud cites a discussion between Antoninus and Rabbi Yehuda HaNasi concerning the precise point in time that the soul is joined to the body. This joining together of the soul and the body is one of the great miracles, as the Rema states in *Orach Chayim* 6: "The joining together of the soul, which is from the heavenly world, with the body, which is from the earthly world, is truly a wondrous miracle."

Since it is impossible for us to understand how the soul is connected with the body, we are certainly unable to determine with certainty the exact point in time when the soul departs from the body. In this connection we must follow the only guide we have — the rulings of our holy Torah.

The Creator of the Universe caused the soul of life to pass into the body of the human being. Thus, "Man became a living soul." The Meiri, in his commentary on Tractate *Yoma*, refers to a case where an avalanche of stones fell on a poor Jewish victim who was almost completely buried. The Torah tells us that all the laws of the Torah may be violated in order to save the victim's life, "even though it is clear that he cannot possibly live even an hour longer." The Meiri states that even an hour of life has the potential for the eternal life promised to the people of Israel, for in that hour a man may repent of his wrongdoings.

What is the essential nature of life?

In his introduction to the second part of *Guide to the Perplexed*, the Rambam states that any body which possesses self-generated movement may be described as "alive." This refers to any body that can move by itself without help from another source.

Can the ability to move be regarded as an adequate definition of the true nature and holy quality of "life"? Rashi (*Kiddushin* 72) explains a verse in the Book of Iyov by stating that

Hashem says to the human being: "Why should man complain about all the troubles that come upon him? He should remember My great kindnesses to him, since I have given him Life, and not Death." If the definition of life is only "the ability to move," what are these great kindnesses which outweigh all the suffering encountered in life?

However, that same verse with which we started our discussion — if a man carries out the commandments of Hashem, "they will bring him life" — also reveals the essential nature of life. The "life" of a Jew is only true "life" when he uses it in order to perform the commandments of Hashem.

An incident related in the Talmud illustrates this point that, for a Jew, the essence of "life" means only the performance of the commandments of the Torah. The Talmud tells us that there was a period in Jewish history when non-Jewish rulers in the land of Israel forbade the study of the Torah on pain of death. Papus ben Yehudah was amazed to see Rabbi Akiva gather together large numbers of Jews and study the Torah with them in spite of the decree. He asked Rabbi Akiva: "Are you not afraid of the decree?" Rabbi Akiva replied: "If we are afraid when we are engaged in the study of the Torah, which is 'our life and length of days,' how much more so should we be afraid if we stop studying the Torah?" Rabbi Akiva compared the Jewish people to fish in a stream. As long as they remain in the stream, they live. If they are taken out of the stream to dry land, they die. The Torah is compared to water. As long as the Jewish people study the Torah, they are like fish in a stream. As soon as the Jewish people stop studying the Torah, they cannot breathe, like fish on dry land. Thus the essence of life for the Jew is the study and performance of the commandments of the Torah.

There is a law in the Torah which states that if a student is exiled to a "city of refuge" because he accidentally killed a person, the Rabbi who teaches him should also be exiled with him.

The Rambam explains this law in the following manner: "The Torah states that the exile shall 'live' in the city of refuge. This means that he should be given every opportunity to lead a full life. A student who is unable to study the Torah is to be regarded as being dead, and not 'alive.' Therefore, his Rabbi should go into exile with him so that he can continue to study the Torah in exile." This illustrates again that for the Jew the essence of life is the study and observance of the commandments of the Torah.

We can now understand what the Meiri tells us — that we may violate the Laws of the Torah in order to save the life of a Jew even if it is clear that the Jew can only live for one more hour, since in that hour he can repent and acquire eternal life.

Use of Disposable Diapers and Adhesive Plasters on the Sabbath

HaRav Chayim Pinchus Scheinberg,
Rosh Yeshiva, Yeshivas Torah Ohr, Jerusalem;
Rav of Mattersdorf, Jerusalem

Excerpts from an article in "Pathways in Medicine" 7 (Elul 5745-September 1985).

Summary: Rabbi Scheinberg notes Rabbinical opinions which state that on the Sabbath it is forbidden to remove the coverings over the adhesive tabs on disposable diapers and that it is also forbidden to tear off the adhesive tabs from the back of the diaper in order to remove it from the baby before throwing the diaper away. According to these opinions, it is also forbidden to remove the backing of an adhesive bandage (plaster or Band-Aid) on the Sabbath. Rabbi Scheinberg rules that all these actions are, in fact, permissible on the Sabbath: since these attachments cannot be regarded as "permanent," they can therefore be detached on the Sabbath.

I refer to the use of disposable diapers on the Sabbath. I have seen this problem discussed in a new edition of a work which quotes leading Rabbis. I do not agree with the conclusions stated in this work concerning the use of disposable diapers on the Sabbath.

The work refers to a type of disposable diaper called "Snugglers." These have two plastic tabs which extend from the two edges of the rear portion of the diaper. These tabs are covered by a strip of plastic which has to be removed before the diaper is placed on the infant. When the plastic covering is removed, the tabs are seen to be covered by a strong glue. After the diaper has been fitted around the baby, the ends of the tabs are glued to the other end of the diaper, securing it firmly around the baby. After half an hour, the glue becomes very firm and it becomes almost impossible to remove the tabs without tearing the diaper. An hour or two later, when the diaper is usually removed, these tabs are torn away from the diaper, which is then thrown away.

The author of the work mentioned above first asks if it is permitted to remove the plastic material which covers the two tabs and thus uncover the glue on the tabs. The question is whether the removal of the cover on the plastic tabs should be considered "tearing," which is forbidden on Sabbath. The *Shulchan Aruch* states that glueing paper or leather to the spine of a book is regarded as a form of "sewing," which is forbidden on the Sabbath. Similarly, a person who separates glued pieces of paper or strips of leather from the spine of a book is performing an action which is classified as "tearing." In our case, the removal of the plastic covers from the tabs in order to use the diaper appears to be similar to tearing.

Second, we may ask if we may remove the adhesive tabs from the back of the diaper before disposing of the diaper. If the attachment of the adhesive tabs to the back of the diaper is regarded as permanent, it could be comparable to a "permanent knot," which may not be untied on the Sabbath. If this is so, it would not be permitted to tear off the adhesive tabs on the

Sabbath before throwing away the diaper. An attachment or a knot, which is not intended to hold or last can be undone or untied on the Sabbath. Thus, if the glued attachment is, in fact, to be regarded as a temporary or "impermanent," it would be permitted to detach the tabs from the diaper on the Sabbath.

In respect to the above, the author of the book referred to is of the opinion that the sticking of the tab to the diaper is permanent. He reasons that after use the diaper is torn open and thrown away, but the adhesive tab usually remains in position. The glue is so strong that it's very difficult to detach the tabs.

With reference to the plastic material that covers the adhesive tabs, the author states that it is clear that this cover is intended to remain on the tab from the day the diaper is produced in the factory until the moment of use. There is a Rabbinical opinion that a knot which is not intended to be permanent, but in fact *stays in place* for a reasonable length of time, should be regarded as a permanent knot and may not be tied or untied on the Sabbath. The Mordechai states that a knot which can stay in place for more than seven days should be regarded as a permanent knot, while other Rabbinical authorities maintain that even a knot that is intended to last only one day should be considered permanent. Thus, in the case of the removal of the cover of the glued plastic tab of the diaper, the author argues, it should also be regarded as a permanent attachment, in which case its removal would be forbidden on the Sabbath.

There is a contrary opinion which maintains that knots should only be considered permanent if there is no intention at all to undo them for a reasonable time, but if there is a possibility that the knot will be untied after a short time, it should not be considered permanent. The example given is sealed vessels of preserved fruit. Although the seal is made to remain in position for a long time, sometimes the seal is broken open after only a short time in order to remove the fruit; it, therefore, is not regarded as permanent and can be broken open on the Sabbath.

The author, however, is of the opinion that this distinction is not applicable to the case we are discussing. He states that the covers are placed on the adhesive tabs in the factory, where vast numbers of diapers are produced for sale, perhaps all over the world, and there is virtually no possibility that the covers on the tabs will be removed within a few days. It could take six months or longer before the diaper reaches the purchaser, which is why the cover on the tabs must be regarded as permanent.

The author gives another reason for forbidding the removal of the backing from adhesive bandages (Band-Aids) or the covering on the adhesive tabs of the diaper on the Sabbath. He states that it may well be that the removal of the backing from the adhesive bandage or the removal of the covering from the adhesive tab on the diaper could be regarded as a "final hammer blow," an act which is forbidden on the Sabbath. The bandage or the diaper is not ready for use until the backing or covering material has been removed. Thus, the removal of the backing or the covering material may be regarded as the final hammer blow which completes the work and makes the bandage or diaper available for use.

With reference to the question of whether or not it is permitted to pull the adhesive tabs off the ends of the diaper before throwing it away, one could say that when the mother stuck the tabs down, she did not intend them to be permanently attached to the diaper. On the contrary, she had every intention of removing them in another hour or two when she changed the baby. Thus it would appear that it would be permitted to tear off the adhesive tabs from the diaper on the Sabbath. The author, however, adopts the view of other Rabbis who maintain that it is not possible to take into account the intention of the person tying the knot. He is of the opinion that in such cases we only consider the nature of the knot, not the intention of the person tying. If a knot is tied so strongly that it will clearly remain in place for some time, it must be regarded as a permanent knot, even if there is a possibility that someone will decide to undo it within a short time.

In fact, the author points out, mothers do not even try to separate the adhesive tab from the diaper when they change the baby, but merely tear the diaper. The glued attachment of the tab to the diaper must be regarded as permanent.

The author concludes that the material covering the adhesive tab of the diaper must not be removed on the Sabbath. It must be regarded as permanent and to remove it would be equivalent to untying a permanent knot on the Sabbath, which is forbidden. Similarly, the attachment of the tab to the diaper is permanent and must not be torn apart on the Sabbath.

In conclusion, the author rules that the only way to use this type of disposal diaper on the Sabbath is with safety-pins, in the same way that they are used with ordinary cloth diapers. The cover should not be removed from the tabs at all.

I do not agree with this ruling. In my opinion, the attachments referred to are not comparable to a permanent knot, but are in fact temporary or impermanent attachments which may be removed on the Sabbath.

In my opinion, the removal of the covering from the adhesive tabs and the removal of the backing from the adhesive bandage are identical to the removal of seals from bottles of fruit, which is permissible on the Sabbath. Even though the seals were intended to last a long time, in order to preserve the fruit, in fact, they are often opened after a short time and cannot be regarded as permanent.

We may find support for my view from the knots that the Children of Israel tied in order to secure their tents while they were journeying through the desert. They are described in the Talmud as knots which were temporary — *not* permanent. However, it is known that the Children of Israel dismantled their tents only when instructed to do so through the command of Hashem. Sometimes they did not move from an encampment for a year, or even two. The knots are nevertheless regarded as impermanent because they never knew when they would be ordered to undo them. Sometimes they had to be undone after only a few hours.

It appears to me that a permanent knot is one that is tied with the *intention* that it should remain fastened permanently. An "impermanent" knot is one which is tied with the intention that it be undone whenever required. In the cases we have been discussing, the attachment is not intended to be permanent, but to be detached when the diaper or the adhesive bandage is needed. The only reason they have not been detached yet is that the moment has not yet arrived for making use of the diaper or bandage. As the attachments have not been made for any fixed period of time, they must be regarded as impermanent and may, therefore, be detached on the Sabbath. In this respect they are comparable to the seals on the bottles of preserved fruit, which are also not regarded as permanent. Even if the attachment is not detached within a day, since it can be detached at any moment — whenever the diaper or plaster is needed — it cannot be described as permanent.

The attachment of the backing to the adhesive bandage and the covering to the adhesive tabs, are not comparable to knots at all, except in a technical sense. They are by their nature impermanent coverings which are intended to be removed as soon as the plaster or diaper is needed. Again, in the case of the tabs glued to the back of the diaper, the mother has no desire, or intention, for the attachment to be permanent. On the contrary, she expects it to be impermanent, so she can make use of the diaper and then throw it away.

One may compare this to the case of an oven which has had its opening closed up by a partition in order to keep the food in it warm. There, it is permitted to remove the partition from the oven opening on the Sabbath for the purpose of removing the food, even if the partition has been very firmly sealed to the oven. The sealed partition is by its very nature permanent, since it was attached strongly. Nevertheless, since its purpose was only to keep the food in the oven warm, and the food was to be removed when needed, it is not to be regarded as a permanent attachment. It is in no way comparable to a permanent knot and may be removed from the oven on the Sabbath.

In my opinion, the material covering the tabs of the diaper and the backing covering the adhesive bandage are not comparable to permanent knots at all, but are merely coverings intended to be removed when necessary. Similarly, the attachment of the tab to the diaper is not a permanent attachment; when the mother glues the tabs down, she only does so with the express intention of tearing them off again an hour or so later when the diaper is no longer needed.

Since they are not comparable to permanent knots, it is permissible to remove the coverings and break the attachments on the Sabbath.

Conclusion: In my opinion, it is permissible on the Sabbath to remove the cover from the adhesive tabs on the disposal diaper and to detach the adhesive tabs from the diaper after use in order to take a diaper off a baby, contrary to the opinion referred to above.

Laniado Hospital as a Torah Institution

Rabbi Moshe Feinstein, of Blessed Memory, Rosh Yeshiva, Mesivta Tifereth Yerushalayim, New York

This is from an article in "Pathways in Medicine" 3-4 (Av 5740 — July 1980).

Summary: In this article, the Gaon, the late Rabbi Moshe Feinstein, of blessed memory, recalls his delight when he heard about the founding of the Laniado Hospital, and calls on all Jewish people to generously support this institutio.

I have heard about the wonderful works carried out in the Holy Land by the saintly Gaon, the Admor of Sanz, the Klausenberger Rabbi, *ztz"l*, and how he has established an Orthodox hospital, the Laniado Hospital in Kiryat Sanz, Netanya. This will be a boon to sick people, who will receive treatment in accordance with the Laws of the Torah. There is great merit in building a hospital for Jewish people which will save the lives of so many and is so desperately needed in the whole region. Apart from this, there is even greater value to a hospital such as Laniado that has been established as a Torah institution, administered by religious, God-fearing people and guided by Rabbis who instruct the staff so they can follow every minute detail of Jewish Law, and which is led by the saintly Gaon, the Admor of Sanz, the Klausenberger Rav, *ztz"l*. These rabbis guard the sanctity of kashrut and the Sabbath in the institution. They have, for example, arranged that none of the nurses or hospital staff will travel on the holy Sabbath. All the arrangements in the Hospital are thus in conformity with the Torah, which is indeed a source of great rejoicing to all God-fearing and religious people. It is impossible to measure the devotion and selfless service to the Torah which this hospital in the Land of Israel exemplifies.

It is indeed a very holy and meritorious deed to support this hospital with contributions on a level suitable to the great needs of this holy project, so it may develop, progress and carry out all its objectives without being hindered by lack of finance. We must understand that this is indeed a lifesaving project. I was, therefore especially delighted to hear that there are plans to build an additional wing to the hospital, and so it is up to all our Jewish brethren to extend a generous hand in this vital matter. If we do this, Hashem will surely fulfil His promises and will remove sickness from among our people.

Five Medical Topics

Rabbi Moshe Feinstein, of Blessed Memory,
Rosh Yeshiva, Mesivta Tifereth Yerushalayim,
New York

Excerpts from articles in "Pathways in Medicine" 6 (Sivan 5744 — June 1985).

Rabbi Feinstein discusses five medical problems in the light of the rulings of the Torah.

1. How should doctors and the nursing staff treat a dying patient?

Summary: Rabbi Feinstein emphasizes that a dying patient should not be touched in any way. He also states that when a dying patient is suffering greatly, the doctor is not obligated to administer life-prolonging drugs if he feels that they will not be effective, but will only increase the patient's suffering.

The Talmud (*Kesubos* 104) relates an account of Rabbi Yehudah HaNasi (Rebbi). When he was critically ill, the Rabbis prayed for his recovery. They felt that as a result of their prayers, his sufferings would be alleviated, but their prayers had not been accepted, and it was clear that he would soon die. When Rebbi's maidservant realised this situation, she prayed that he die quickly. Rebbi's maidservant was recognized as a great Torah scholar in her own right, and the Rabbis listened to her views. We may therefore learn from her example that one is permitted to pray for the early death of a person who is suffering greatly if there is no chance that he will survive. Again, in *Maseches Nedarim* 40 we find the opinion of Rabbi Dimi that a person who does not wish to visit a sick man will neither pray for his survival, nor for *his early death*. From this statement of Rabbi Dimi, the Ran concludes that there are times when one is permitted to pray for the early death of a sick person, such as when he is suffering greatly and there is almost no chance he will survive.

From this we may conclude that if a patient is so critically ill that experts feel that there is virtually no hope that he will live, and, moreover, he is suffering greatly because of his illness, a doctor may, if he thinks fit, *refrain* from administering life-preserving drugs and stop all treatment. He must not, however, take any action which could *shorten* the patient's life by even one second: this is considered by the Torah as equivalent to murder. Again, if it is possible to administer a drug which would alleviate the patient's suffering, but would not shorten his life in any way, such drugs *must* be administered.

Thus a dying patient who has difficulty in breathing should be given oxygen, as difficulty in breathing causes great suffering, and administering oxygen eases breathing and consequently alleviates suffering. However, care should be taken that the patient receives oxygen say for an hour or two, and then is carefully observed before being given more oxygen. If he is still suffering, then oxygen should be given for another hour or two and then the patient observed again. In this way the danger of causing the patient's death through negligence can be averted, and the patient will receive constant care, so his life may be prolonged, even for an extra second.

I have heard some doctors are not careful to note the exact moment when a dying patient has entered his last phase of life, and they are not aware of the importance of not touching a patient during the last moments of life, as we are commanded in the Torah. It may be that non-Jewish doctors are not aware of the importance of this prohibition, or it may be that they are aware of it, but do not concern themselves too much with it. There are many proofs from the Torah that a non-Jew as well as a Jew is forbidden to touch a patient during the last phase of the patient's life, in case, by so doing, he brings his death nearer, which is classified as a form of murder. Many non-Jewish doctors are not particular about this, and even some non-observant Jewish doctors touch dying patients; either they do not know better, or they do not care. Orthodox Jews should endeavor to be present when a Jewish patient is dying in their hospital, to assist the Rabbis of the Burial Society and to ensure that the patient is treated in the manner required by the Laws of the Torah.

2. "Sterilisation after sterilisation"

Summary: Rabbi Feinstein states that if a patient is undergoing an operation for removal of the womb, the ovaries and fallopian tubes may also be removed at the same time, even though they may be healthy, in order to avoid the risk of cancer at a later date. However, the patient and her husband should be consulted first, and the opinion of a religious doctor obtained.

When they perform an operation to remove a womb, surgeons also frequently remove the ovaries and the fallopian tubes, even though they may be perfectly healthy. They state that they do this because there is five per cent chance that the ovaries and the fallopian tubes may at some later date become affected by cancer, and as they are already operating, they consider it advisable to take advantage of the situation and remove the ovaries and fallopian tubes at the same time. I have been asked if this procedure is forbidden according to Jewish law, which forbids unnecessary sterilisation. In this case, it is clear that there is no question of sterilisation; the removal of the womb has rendered the patient incapable of having children in any case. Similarly, we learn in Tractate *Shabbos* 111 that a woman who is incapable of having children is permitted to drink a medicine which has the effect of sterilisation, as she cannot have children in any case; this may be classified as "sterilisation after sterilisation," which would not be forbidden here. In the case we are discussing, since the surgeons are compelled to remove the diseased womb, there is no reason why they should not also remove the ovaries and fallopian tubes. Even though there is only a five percent chance that cancer will develop in the ovaries and the fallopian tubes, it must be considered a dangerous risk.

This is true even though we maintain that a person should only undergo an operation if there is at least a twenty per cent risk, or more, that he may die without it, because an operation is in itself a risky procedure which should not be undertaken lightly. In this case, the operation is already being performed, and we may assume that no extra suffering will be caused to the patient if the surgeon extends the operation. In fact, the additional surgery may even give the patient greater comfort after the operation. The patient and her husband should be asked if they agree, and the opinion of a religious doctor should also be obtained before it is done.

3. Should a patient who refuses to take a medicine prescribed by a doctor be compelled to take it against his will?

Summary: Rabbi Feinstein states that it is permissible to force a patient to take a medicine if there is no good reason for his refusal and on condition that the patient will not become frightened by being forced. He adds that if the medicine itself could cause some harm in some circumstances, a patient should never be forced to take it.

If a patient does not wish to take medicine for reasons which appear to be childish, e.g., he does not like the taste or does not wish to be disturbed, even though he believes that the doctor is responsible and is prescribing the correct medicine for him, he may be compelled to take the medicine. However, if the patient refuses to take the medicine because he does not trust the particular doctor who prescribed it, then, if possible, another doctor should be found whom the patient does trust. If no such doctor can be found, or if there is no time to find another doctor due to the urgency of the situation, then the doctor, in consultation with and with the agreement of the other doctors in the hospital, should try to compel the patient to take the medicine. However, if there is a risk that the patient may become terrified or shocked if he is compelled to take the medicine, he should not be forced to take it, even if his refusal is only for childish reasons; his fear may cause his condition to deteriorate and may even cause earlier death. If the medicine itself may cause some harm, and the doctors normally balance the risk of it causing harm against the seriousness of the illness, and the person refuses to take it, he should not be compelled in any way to take it.

4. Abortions are strictly forbidden

Summary: Rabbi Feinstein states that abortions are regarded by Jewish Law as a form of murder, unless they are declared to be necessary in order to protect the health of the mother. He reminds us that this prohibition applies to non-Jewish mothers as well as Jewish mothers, and that no assistance should be given to any form of prohibited abortion.

In our troubled times, there are misguided mothers who wrongly ask doctors to abort their unborn child in the womb. Such an action is strictly forbidden and must be regarded as a form of murder. It is also forbidden to assist the performance of such abortions in any way. This prohibition applies to non-Jewish mothers as well as Jewish mothers, since, according to the Torah, non-Jews are also forbidden to murder, which includes the killing of the unborn child in the womb. One need not be concerned that refusing to help a non-Jewish mother abort her child will cause hatred of Jewish people. A God-fearing Jewish doctor can explain to the non-Jewish mother that he does not wish to assist in the destruction of a child in the womb, for the child is regarded as a human being — unless it is absolutely necessary for the health of the mother. It is likely that the non-Jewish mother will understand his point of view, which is even upheld by the laws of certain countries.

5. Operation to relieve suffering of cancer patient

Summary: Rabbi Feinstein states that it is permissible to operate on a patient suffering from incurable cancer with the intention of relieving his suffering, even if he will be sterilised as a result of the operation.

I have been asked if an operation to remove a cancerous portion of the body (the prostate, which may also involve the removal of testicles) is permissible in the case of a patient who has widespread cancer that is incurable in the opinion of the specialists. The operation is not intended to cure the patient, which is considered impossible, but merely to alleviate the pain and suffering felt by the patient as a result of this incurable disease. This operation is clearly permissible; an operation may be carried out in order to alleviate the suffering of a seriously ill patient. Also, such an operation may prolong the life of a patient. It is well known that if two patients are suffering from the same disease, one in pain and the other free from pain, the patient free from pain usually lives longer. Pain itself can cause a speedier death.

Thus, the operation referred to is permissible even if it results in the sterilisation of the patient, since the patient is critically ill, and the operation will relieve his suffering.

Use of a Digital Contact Thermometer on the Sabbath

HaRav Eliezer Yehuda Waldenberg,
Chief Dayan, Rabbinical Court of Jerusalem

Excerpts from an article in "Pathways in Medicine" 1 (Adar 5739 — March 1979).

Summary: Rabbi Waldenberg discusses whether or not it is permissible to use digital contact thermometers on the Sabbath. These are strips of film which are placed on the forehead of the patient. If the patient has a temperature, certain letters or colours appear on the film. Rabbi Waldenberg concludes that it is permissible to use such thermometers on the Sabbath.

I have been asked if a new type of thermometer, called *Galei HaChom*, which is now available in Israel, may be used on the Sabbath. This thermometer consists of a thin, filmlike ribbon which is closely applied to the forehead of the patient. After a few seconds, if the patient has a normal temperature, the letter *N* appears on the film. If the patient's temperature is 37-38 degrees centigrade, the letters *NF* appear on the film. If the temperature is higher than 38 degrees centigrade, only the letter *F* appears.

I have seen a related problem is discussed by the Pri Megadim on *Orach Chayim* 34:7. The Pri Megadim writes: "A person wishes to write a secret message. He writes the message on paper with unboiled milk instead of ink. A second person receives the paper with the message written on it and warms it up before a flame. The message becomes visible. If this is done on the Sabbath, the second person is not liable for a sin offering for violating the Sabbath. However, the Rabbis have decreed that this heating-up action should not be performed on the Sabbath because it resembles 'writing.' "

At first sight, the question of the digital contact thermometer seems to be similar to the question raised by the Pri Megadim. The letters indicating the temperature are made visible by the body heat of the patient, just as the secret writing appears on the paper when it is heated by the flame. The same law could be said to apply. The use of the digital contact thermometer on the Sabbath would not be a Biblical violation of the Sabbath, but would nevertheless be forbidden by Rabbinical decree.

Moreover, a case found in the Jerusalem Talmud (*Shabbos* chap. 12) appears to suggest that the use of the digital contact thermometer could even be forbidden on the Sabbath by Biblical law. The Jerusalem Talmud describes a case where a person wishes to write a secret message. He writes the message on paper without using ink; he merely makes indentations in the paper with a pen. The person who receives the message then carefully fills in the indentations with ink so the writing becomes visible. The Rabbis in the Jerusalem Talmud declare that this would be forbidden on the Sabbath by Biblical Law, not merely by Rabbinical decree, as it is equivalent to "writing." From this it would appear that the use of the digital contact thermometer on the Sabbath could also be forbidden by Biblical Law.

On closer examination, however, one can see that the two

cases are not exactly the same. In the case quoted in the Jerusalem Talmud, the person receiving the message actually uses a writing material, namely ink, to make the letters visible. In the case described by the Pri Megadim, actual writing material is not used by the second person. The paper with the letters written on it in milk is heated, which makes the letters appear. Therefore, it is reasonable to assume that in the case described in the Jerusalem Talmud, the act would be forbidden by Biblical law, whereas in the case quoted by the Pri Megadim the act would be forbidden by Rabbinical decree. Clearly, the Pri Megadim must have known the ruling of the Jerusalem Talmud when he came to his decision about heating the letters written with milk. It is reasonable to assume that were it not for the case quoted by the Jerusalem Talmud, the Pri Megadim might have come to the conclusion that the case he was considering would not be forbidden at all, even by Rabbinical decree. Such a consideration would make it easier to permit the use of the digital contact thermometer on the Sabbath, where, for various reasons, the situation is even less stringent than the case of heating letters written in milk, as we will see.

Another case is quoted in the *Shulchan Aruch* which is similar to the case of the digital contact thermometer. Some Rabbis rule that if wax falls on writing, obscuring some of the letters, it is forbidden to remove the wax on the Sabbath, because by doing so, one, as it were, "rewrites" the covered letters. The Bach states that if two letters are made visible by removing the wax, then a Biblical prohibition has been violated, but if only one letter is made visible, a Rabbinical decree has been broken. The Pri Megadim does not agree with this ruling; he claims that such an action should not be classed as "writing" at all, since one has not written anything new by removing the wax — the letters already existed. He does agree that the person should not have touched the wax on the Sabbath, as such an action is forbidden by the Rabbis because the wax is *muktzeh*.

One may conclude from the case of the wax obscuring the letters — which, according to the Pri Megadim is not to be classed as "writing" — that the use of the digital contact thermometer should also not be classed as "writing": the letters already existed, and they were merely "uncovered" by the heat of the body temperature.

Moreover, in the case of the digital contact thermometer, it is possible that all Rabbis would agree that its use on the Sabbath would not be forbidden, even by Rabbinical decree. The letters appear on the film only briefly, and as soon as the film is removed from the forehead of the patient, they disappear. Thus, there is even less reason to compare the letters to "writing." This may be compared to another case mentioned by our Rabbis which is also not to be considered "writing." The question arose as to whether or not it is permitted to open a book if a person had written words on the edges of the pages; if the book was opened and then closed on the Sabbath, the writing would reappear. The Rabbis decided that such an action is permissible on the Sabbath, because the writing does not endure; it is not permanent and, therefore, cannot be considered to be "writing." Similarly, the letters which appear on the film of the digital contact thermometer do not remain in place for more than a minute or two, and cannot be considered "writing." For all these reasons, one could conclude that the digital contact thermometer may be used on the Sabbath.

The problem of erasing in the case of the digital contact thermometer

One might claim that a problem arises when the thermometer is removed from the patient's head. The letters then disappear, which could be regarded as "erasing" writing, which is forbidden on the Sabbath. In addition, this erasing lasts for some time. Unlike the "writing" of the letters of the thermometer, which only remains visible for a short time, the letters remain erased out until the thermometer is used again, which could be hours or even days later.

This argument, however, can be shown not to be a valid one. The so-called "erasing" is not really erasing in the full meaning of the expression as concerns the laws of Sabbath, which are based on work performed by the Children of Israel when they constructed the Tabernacle in the wilderness. In the work on the Tabernacle, there was no erasing that could be restored immediately, as with the digital contact thermometer. Thus, there is no reason to prohibit the use of the digital contact thermometer on the Sabbath because of the prohibition against erasing because the letters can be restored without any difficulty.

There is another vital factor to be considered in the case of a digital contact thermometer. This thermometer is not normally used for healthy people, but for ill patients, and especially for ill children. They may not be seriously ill, but the thermometer is used to ascertain whether they are. As we have seen, this discussion is centered only on whether or not the thermometer is forbidden in Rabbinical law. All agree that it is permissible in Biblical Law. Therefore, because we are considering cases of illness, which could be serious, there is no reason at all to prohibit the use of such a thermometer on the Sabbath.

From all we have considered above, it appears that it is permissible to use the digital contact thermometer on the Sabbath for persons who are not feeling well, especially where it is difficult to use a regular thermometer, as with children.

The digital contact colour thermometer

I have also been asked about another type of thermometer similar to the one we have been discussing. This works on the same principle, except that the letters change colours when the patient has a temperature. As the temperature increases, the letters shine with a deeper and deeper green. The question is asked, may this thermometer be used on the Sabbath, for since the letters become a deeper green, this could be classified as a form of "painting" or "colouring," forbidden on the Sabbath. Again, this does not appear to be a reason for prohibiting the use of such a thermometer on the Sabbath. The colour which appears does not last — it disappears as soon as the thermometer is removed from the patient — and therefore should not be considered "colouring" according to the Laws of the Sabbath.

There is another reason that allows us to be lenient. The Torah tells us that the colouring must cover an area of at least four *tefachim* (handbreadths) before it can be regarded as colouring, and the letters on the thermometer are far smaller. Incidentally, this is the reason I ruled elsewhere that spots of urine on a board may be coloured in order to carry out certain tests on the Sabbath — they are not big enough to fall within the category of "colouring."

In addition, the change of colour on the thermometer is not actually colouring, but is rather a weakening or intensification of colours that already exist in the thermometer. Rabbi Moshe

Feinstein, of blessed memory, was once asked if it is permissible to wear a new type of sunglasses on the Sabbath, which automatically darken when the wearer enters strong sunlight and lighten in the shade. He replied that he could see no connection between this and the prohibition of colouring on the Sabbath, as the colours are already present in the glass. He ruled that such glasses could be worn on the Sabbath, and the same reasoning applies to the type of digital contact thermometer which we have been discussing. In our case, the heat brings out the colour, and the removal of the heat takes away the colour that is already in the film, just like the case of the sunglasses where the bright light brings out the darker colours in the glass and the weaker light removes them.

Thus I conclude that both types of digital contact thermometers may be used on the Sabbath.

"Family Planning" according to Jewish Law

HaRav Yaakov Landau,
Rav of Bnei Brak

Excerpts from an article in "Pathways in Medicine" 1 (Adar 5739 — March 1979).

Summary: Rabbi Landau warns Jewish women against the false advice of so-called "experts" who recommend the use of "family planning" methods in order to limit the size of their families. He states that such methods are contrary to Jewish Law, except in special cases where authority has been obtained from a qualified and experienced Rabbi.

The blessing which the Almighty gave to our father Avraham — "And I will cause you to multiply greatly" — has been the symbol and foundation of Jewish family life throughout the history of our people wherever we have lived, even in exile from our land. As it says in Tehillim 127: "Lo, children are a heritage of the Lord; the fruit of the womb is a reward. As arrows in the hand of a mighty man, so are the children of one's youth. Happy is the man that has his quiver full of them." As the great Rabbinical commentator known as the Radak explained: the greatest reward that the Almighty can give in this world to those who love Him is children.

And we find in Tehillim 128: "Thy wife shall be as a fruitful vine, in the innermost parts of thy house. Thy children shall be like olive plants round about thy table." The Alshich explains this verse in the following manner: Just as one sees on a vine both small and large grapes, so the family which has been blessed by the Almighty will have older children and younger children all together at the same time in the family. Our great Rabbis have stated that this is a blessing for which every truly religious man should pray.

Throughout our history, the Jewish people have always made great sacrifices in order to have large families. Even when the Children of Israel were in Egypt, suffering beneath the oppression of Pharaoh, Jewish mothers made great sacrifices in order to fulfil the commandment to have large families. The biblical commentators tell us that the father of Moshe separated himself completely from his wife when he heard the terrible decree of Pharaoh: "Every male Jewish baby shall be drowned in the Nile." They relate that the sister of Moshe, the prophetess Miriam, said to her father: "Your decree is worse than the decree of Pharaoh. Pharaoh has passed a decree against male infants. You are passing a decree against male *and* female infants." As a result of Miriam's words, Moshe's father reunited with his wife, and Miriam's plea — a plea against "family restriction" — resulted in the birth of our great leader and saviour, Moshe, who led the Jewish people out of Egypt.

So it was, throughout our history, even during times of the greatest poverty and difficulty, that the women of Israel flourished like "vines," as the Psalmist says. They put their trust in the Creator of Life who also brings sustenance to the world. As our Rabbis state (*Niddah* 31): "When a baby boy is born, he arrives with a loaf of bread in his hands!"

The Torah tells us that Pharaoh said that he passed his decree against the Children of Israel "in case they should multiply." The commentators tell us at that moment a voice came down from Heaven and cried out to Pharaoh: "And indeed they will multiply! The more you persecute them, the more they will flourish!"

And now, in modern times, so-called "experts," who are themselves Jewish, acting in official capacities, try to persuade Jewish women to despise the blessings of the Almighty and limit the size of their families. I am referring to certain organisations which have lately begun a treacherous campaign among our people. They do all they can to persuade Jewish women to use so-called family planning methods. They appoint special doctors to advise Jewish women to follow these methods. They even open special clinics to supply and fit women with family planning devices. Some even visit the homes of families where there are already two children and use all kinds of professional talk to persuade parents not to have any more children, emphasizing all the while that they are only acting for the good of the family and the community.

To my sorrow I have even heard that doctors have advised religious mothers that there is no restriction on family planning according to Jewish Law. They claim that, according to the Torah, a woman has no obligation to have a family. They even quote the holy *Shulchan Aruch,* where it mentions that a Jewish woman is permitted to drink a certain drug that will stop her from having children. The truth is that this statement refers only to a case where a woman has severe problems in childbirth. In fact the Chasam Sofer wrote that, in his opinion, a married woman is not permitted to drink the contraceptive drug mentioned in the *Shulchan Aruch.* Also, it must be pointed out that this section in the *Shulchan Aruch* refers only to drinking a drug, not to the insertion of a contraceptive device in the mother's womb, which in fact entails another serious prohibition. It is not permissible for a man to emit semen except to conceive and have children, and thus, if such a device has been fitted, the husband, in fact, will be liable of committing the sin of emitting and destroying semen that cannot cause conception, a serious transgression according to Jewish Law. If the husband knows that this is forbidden and still ignores the prohibition, his punishment is most severe according to Jewish Law.

The prohibition against the use of family planning does not apply to special cases where permission has been given by a qualified Rabbi

It should be made clear that all I have stated above refers to normal cases. There are special cases according to Jewish Law, where contraceptive methods *should* be used. These are cases where the persons concerned have received permission from a highly trained, experienced and fully qualified Rabbi.

There is another very important point that requires emphasis. The use of contraceptives without permission from a Rabbi is an attack on the very foundation of our faith. It reveals a lack of belief in the capability of the Almighty to feed and satisfy the needs of all His creatures. It denies that the Almighty exercises detailed and full control over all the workings of the Universe for our own good and it is contrary to the basic tenets of Judaism. Those who practice contraception without Rabbinical permission demonstrate that they believe their well-being is entirely in their own hands and they are in complete control of their fate. They use contraception because they believe incorrectly that they cannot afford to have more children, or simply because it is inconvenient for them to have a large family.

Judaism, however, teaches us that the whole purpose of our creation is only to carry out the wishes of the Almighty, Who is able to satisfy all our needs.

We may bring an illustration from the biblical account of the construction of King Solomon's Temple. Our commentators ask why King Solomon ordered his servants to be away from their homes for only one month at a time and be at home with their wives for two months when he sent them out of Israel to import material for the construction of the Temple. They answer that King Solomon feared if the husbands were away from home for longer than a month at a time, it could result in a diminution of the number of Jewish children born. From this our Rabbis learn that a large number of births in Jewish families is more precious in the eyes of the Almighty than the construction of the Temple!

The Torah teaches us that even if a man already has children, the obligation to have more children still remains with him. We are also taught in the Torah that Moshiach will not come until all the souls in Heaven which have to be born are born. From this we learn in the Talmud that those who have many children are bringing closer the day of the coming of Moshiach.

We issue a call to our righteous Jewish women: Guard your own futures and bring nearer the day of our Redemption! Do not listen to the false advice of those who combine contraception with family planning. Instead, follow in the footsteps of our holy and righteous ancestors!

Psychiatry and Religion

HaRav Shlomo Wolbe, Jerusalem

Excerpts from an article in "Pathways in Medicine" 5 (Sivan 5742 — June 1982).

Summary: Rabbi Wolbe examines certain psychiatric cases and situations from the point of view of the Torah and Jewish Law. He comes to the conclusion that the Torah can contribute greatly to our understanding of psychiatric problems, and that there is room for an ongoing partnership between those learned in Torah and our practising psychiatrists.

The relationship between Orthodox religion and psychiatric treatment

The general approach of the Torah to the practise of medicine is well-known. The doctor is given the full right to heal, as the Torah states: "Thou shalt surely heal" (Shemos 21:19). Also, every person is obligated "to take good care of himself" (Devarim 4:15). Many Rabbis hold the opinion that the duty of a doctor to heal is a Biblical, not Rabbinical, injunction, with all the implied stringencies. It should be understood that psychiatry has the same status, from the point of view of the Torah, as every other branch of medicine. It is quite clear that any serious mental derangement, neurotic or psychotic, should be diagnosed by a psychiatrist and treated by him as soon as possible. Unfortunately, for two reasons, this has not been grasped by the general public. Firstly, there are many preconceived notions about mental illness, and second, there is a prevalant lack of knowledge about all aspects of the subject.

Preconceived notions in connection with mental illness

The most frightening of all the preconceived notions about mental illness is the idea that such illness is a blemish on the whole family. I have witnessed a case where the members of an exceptionally fine family refused to accept the fact that their dear son was suffering from schizophrenia. At first they refused to accept the diagnosis. Then, as the illness progressed, they began to ignore the patient. He left home and stayed in an institution where he received no treatment at all. Any person who has influence on such a family is obligated to try to persuade them to help the patient receive psychiatric treatment — as soon as possible!

A second preconceived notion concerns someone who has received treatment for mental illness in a hospital or other institution. It is incorrectly believed that anyone who has received such treatment is branded for life as an "outsider" and will be excluded from normal society, even after he has been completely cured. The patient's family also often fear that his admission to an institution will make his illness worse.

There is, therefore, a great need to explain to the general public that doctors in the field are well aware of this situation, and they take all possible care to ensure that no patient is admitted to a hospital or institution unless it is absolutely necessary. The general public should also be made aware of the fact that there are now many new drugs at the disposal of psychiatrists which have revolutionised the treatment of mental illness.

Almost every Orthodox Jewish patient who is referred to a psychiatrist or psychologist asks if there is a danger that the treatment he will receive will have a negative effect on his religious faith. If the patient is psychotic, the family should be told that the doctor concerned will treat the patient just as any other doctor would treat a sick person — with medicines and other recognised forms of treatment. However, if the patient is only neurotic, there is, in fact, some risk involved if the psychiatrist treats him in certain conventional psychiatric ways. For instance, if an Orthodox Jewish patient is told that his illness is caused by "repression of his sexual instincts" and that in order to cure himself he must "liberate" his sexual instincts from this "repression," it is likely to cause bitter internal conflict, which could lead to a loss of religious faith and even suicide. A very experienced non-religious psychiatric specialist once confided to me that his conscience would not allow him to accept Orthodox Jewish patients for treatment.

Not only is this kind of medical approach open to criticism, but, sometimes, the psychiatrist himself is not up to high professional standards. A highly intelligent young lady was once referred to me. Her husband was a Rabbi who studied all day in a talmudical college. The lady was physically healthy in every respect, but she complained to me that she had no satisfaction from her life and she was depressed. I advised her to suggest to her husband that he take up a position as a communal Rabbi, for which he was fully qualified. In carrying out her duties as the Rabbi's wife, she would find an outlet for her intellectual talents. The lady had already visited a number of psychiatrists and psychologists, one of whom had advised her to find a "boyfriend." I would consider the capabilities and standards of the psychiatrist who gave her this advice gravely suspect, quite apart from the fact that he was completely lacking in tact. We can well imagine the consequences if the young lady had accepted her psychiatrist's advice. Her strong feelings of guilt would, without doubt, have reduced her to a neurotic condition. Such situations should never be allowed to occur! People working in the field of mental health should be made aware of the fact that the Jewish religious community refuses to have any connection with the modern plague of sexual permissiveness, and we must thank Hashem for His goodness that this is the case. The Orthodox Jewish community is disgusted by such behavior. Nonreligious people believe that sexual permissiveness is a symptom of mental health. We, on the other hand, regard it as an incurable plague that has the power to destroy a nation.

*DRUG ADDICTION, AND HOW IT MAY BE OVERCOME
*EXCESSIVE FEELINGS OF GUILT AND HOW THEY MAY BE AVOIDED

These two problems are generally regarded by psychiatrists as distinct, requiring different forms of treatment.

From the religious point of view however, both problems derive from the same source — an incorrect educational approach.

Drug addiction amongst young people: a failure in education

We have pointed out elsewhere that the intelligence should be used to control and direct all our human powers, with the aim of bringing us closer to Hashem. In modern times, the intelligence no longer performs this function. Instead, it is used as an instrument for acquiring knowledge and technology and bringing about "progress." This has lead to intellectual materialism, and one indirect result of the popularization of psychiatry. When a modern young person wishes to come close to Hashem without the use of his intelligence, as it were through the back door, he tries drugs such as hashish, marijuana and L.S.D. and becomes dependent on them.

Modern culture stands helpless against such plagues. Science has no means to deal with the problem. The only educational institutions which are free from the problem are Jewish talmudical colleges, the yeshivos.

When addiction in the United States assumed epidemic proportions, the United States Department of Education sent out a questionnaire to all institutions of higher education requesting information on the extent of drug addiction in each institution and details of the steps the teaching staff was taking to remedy the situation. The largest talmudical college in the United States, the yeshiva in Lakewood, New Jersey, received this questionnaire. The teaching staff replied that the problem did not exist at their College; not one of their 700 students was addicted to drugs.

The Department of Education then sent an inspector to the College. He asked for an answer to the following question: how could drug addiction not exist at the Lakewood Yeshiva, when, in every other institute of higher education, without exception, the problem had reached massive proportions? The Rabbis of the College explained to the Inspector that the environment was such that it would be inconceivable for one student to become addicted to drugs. It was true, they admitted, there were young religious Jews who had become victims to addiction.

What then was the secret of the success of their College? They explained that the intellectual effort required to study the Torah, the holy influence of these studies, and the strong desire that existed among the students to achieve spiritual perfection, were the factors which made the Yeshiva a fortress which drugs could not breach.

It is also a fact that one does not have to be a full-time student at a talmudical college in order to protect himself from the plague of drug addiction. It may well be that any Jew who participates regularly in Torah classes and study groups will be protected. In fact, Jewish Orthodoxy could contribute to the war against drug addiction simply by organising more and more classes and study groups in Torah subjects.

Guilt feelings of the young

Adolescence is a time when "guilt feelings" are very common. This can especially apply to a religious young person. The Torah regards the wastage of male semen as a grave sin. The majority of young people however, do fall into this trap and cannot escape from it. As a result, they develop guilt feelings. This calls for a sympathetic approach on the part of Rabbis and educators. The Rabbi is not able to forgive sins and certainly cannot permit wrongdoing. He can, however, guide and teach the young person to have more patience with himself. In addition, the young person should be encouraged to associate actively with his peers. In particular he should be introduced to the magnificent treasury which is the Torah. As *Pirkei Avos* states: "Torah combined with a worldly occupation is a good thing, since the effort required for both causes a man to forget sin." One learns from this that the effort of studying the Torah combined with social activity leads to a situation where sin is, as it were, "forgotten" by the student. This is the style of education we adopt. It is true that Torah education requires intensive study. Without such education, there is no escape from feelings of guilt and despondency.

Today we live in a society of sexual permissiveness. Young people need great inner strength not to be influenced. We must thank Hashem that in the Orthodox Jewish community the ideals of family purity and ethical perfection are still maintained. We will never give up these ideals. And as we have said, this requires education. Judaism is inconceivable without education!

The treatment of the dying

Today most patients die in hospitals, not in their homes. This fact has placed squarely before the hospital nursing staff the problem of how to treat a dying patient. The question may be put in another way: how can one prepare a patient for death?

There is another aspect to this problem. Many cases have been reported of patients who have "clinically died," and, as a result of intensive medical treatment, "returned to life." They relate elevated experiences, especially during the period when they were clinically dead. They report that they felt that their personalities were detached bodies without any sense of pain: their intelligence seemed to be without limit, and they had deep feelings of contentment. When the efforts to revive them began to succeed, the personality returned to the body, which was by no means a pleasant experience. They recalled that they were "brought back to life" very much against their will, and at once their pain began again. A professor of neurology, who had such an experience, has written a book about it. Many similar reports have been recorded. There is no doubt of their authenticity.

Such reports compel us to reconsider our attitude towards the dying person. The patient may have a pale countenance, be contorted with pain, suffer perhaps from convulsions and scarcely be able to breathe. Yet all the reports tell us that it is just at that time that the dying person may encounter those exceptionally elevated and pleasurable experiences, quite contrary to what one would conclude from his condition! Those who are treating such a person are obligated to exercise the maximum care and consideration. These facts correspond with the words of Tehillim 104, which deals with such matters. The Talmud tells us that David wrote this Psalm "when he was considering the day of his death" (*Berachos* 10). Our Rabbis explain that a person can only achieve this vision on the "day of his death." At the moment a man is leaving this world, the greatness of Hashem is revealed to him.

Jewish Law states that "a dying man must be regarded as alive in all respects." However, as soon as he loses consciousness, who knows what is in store for him? Certainly the hospital staff must exercise the greatest care in how they treat him at such a time, as Jewish Law ordains: Jewish Law states that it is even forbidden to touch a dying person. As long as the patient is conscious, one must be very careful not to foster in him a feeling that he is considered to be seriously ill. The only approach is to give the patient the feeling that he will continue to live as long as possible.

Conclusions

We have surveyed several questions relating to the subject of "Psychiatry and Jewish Law." It is clear that there is room for further research, and as we analyse other cases, we will see that there is need for a common effort in this field. The Torah of Israel teaches us that wisdom is the "building up" of a human being. Psychiatry is the skill of treating the mentally sick. A joint effort can bring many blessings.

Can an Ambulance Return to Its Station on the Sabbath?

HaRav Israel Zalmanowitz,
former Chief Rabbi of Acco

Excerpts from an article in "Pathways in Medicine" 3 - 4 (Av 5740 — July 1980).

Summary: Rabbi Zalmanowitz concludes that Jewish Law permits an ambulance to return to the ambulance station on the Sabbath after transporting a dangerously ill patient to the hospital. He further concludes that the owner of a private vehicle, who has transported a sick person to the hospital on the Sabbath, is permitted to turn off the engine of his car on arrival. In each case, a separate question should be put to the local Rabbi before this is done.

Question:

Can an ambulance that has transported a dangerously ill patient to the hospital, or to a doctor, on the Sabbath return to the ambulance station to be ready to transport another patient?

Answer:

First we should point out that it appears from the Tosafos (*Pesachim* 46) that a call from a dangerously ill patient is not to be considered a common or usual occurrence for which one must be prepared. From this it might appear that an ambulance which has transported a dangerously ill patient on the Sabbath would not be allowed to drive back to its station on the Sabbath to be ready for another emergency call, as we should not regard such calls as a common or usual occurrence for which we must be prepared.

Under today's conditions, however, emergency calls for ambulances take place so often, that ambulances sometimes travel back and forth, regularly transporting emergency cases. In addition, today there are many maternity cases where mothers need emergency transportation to the hospital. Thus it may well be that under present conditions, an ambulance would be permitted to return to the ambulance station on the Sabbath to be available for other emergency cases.

We learn from other Responsa that if there is no seriously ill patient at the time, it is forbidden to make preparations which involve actions that violate the Sabbath in case a patient becomes seriously ill. For example, it is forbidden to prepare medicines for patients who may become dangerously ill, but in fact are not dangerously ill at the moment. Such preparations may be made only for dangerously ill patients who actually need the treatment, and not for a hypothetical emergency case, which may or may not arise.

This situation can be distinguished from the case we are considering. The hospital staff could possibly have prepared these emergency medicines before the Sabbath. In any case, they don't know precisely what medicines will actually be needed until the patient becomes dangerously ill. In the case we are considering, the ambulance is providing a general service which many types of patients require, and, therefore, perhaps the ambulance would be permitted to return to the station to be prepared for all emergency calls, even if these calls have not occurred yet.

From the above discussion, I believe that Jewish Law would permit an ambulance to return to its station on the Sabbath in order to be prepared for emergency calls. In practice, the hospital should put this question to the Rabbi appointed to supervise its religious affairs.

One question always leads to another. We have been discussing the question of an ambulance which normally works through the day and night transporting dangerously ill patients. We may well ask what would be in the case of a small isolated settlement, where a person is suddenly taken very ill on the Sabbath. Let us assume that there is no ambulance available immediately and one of the inhabitants transports the patient to the hospital in his private car. It may be that in the same settlement there is a pregnant woman who could give birth at any moment, or a sick person who is not dangerously ill at the moment but may become so at any time. In such a situation, is the owner of the car permitted to drive back to the settlement on the Sabbath, in case his car is needed to take another sick person to hospital? This question requires deeper study before a final answer can be given.

Can the engine of the car be turned off on the Sabbath?

Another question arises from this situation. Let us assume that the driver of the private vehicle does not return to the settlement on the Sabbath after transporting the sick patient. Is he allowed to turn off the engine of his car or is he required to let the engine of the car run until all the petrol is used up and the engine stops? It is clear that it is not permissible to violate the Sabbath to avoid a monetary loss under any circumstances.

However, if the driver leaves the car engine running, the engine may be damaged, and he may not be able to use the car to transport another sick patient.

In this connection we may quote another case from the Talmud which speaks of a situation where violent enemies are heard to be approaching a settlement on the Sabbath. A group of settlers leave the village, carrying their weapons, in order to confront the enemy. After the enemy has been defeated, the question arises as to whether or not the villagers can return to their settlement with their weapons, or must they leave them behind, because it is still the Sabbath. If they do return without their weapons, there is a risk that they might be attacked by other enemies while they are defenseless. In such a case, they would be allowed to carry their weapons back. There is another consideration. If the villagers were not allowed to carry their weapons back to the settlement, and the same problem arose again, it could be difficult to find volunteers who would go out on the Sabbath to fight marauders: they would assume that they would have to leave their weapons behind when the fight was over and could be attacked by other enemies on the way back. This is comparable to the situation we are discussing: If the driver was compelled to leave his engine running and runs the risk of damaging it, it is very likely that owners of private vehicles in the settlement would be unwilling to transport sick people to the hospital on the Sabbath.

It should be noted that these two cases are not exactly comparable. Carrying the weapons results from a danger to life. Allowing the car engine to run only involves a possible financial loss, which must be balanced against the need to save a sick person's life. While it may be permissible to carry weapons, it may not be possible to conclude from this that a car engine may be turned off on the Sabbath.

However, after making enquiries from car-owners, I learned that if a car engine is left to run for a long time, there is a real risk that it could release the brakes of the car, which could then begin to move forward without a driver. It appears that such occurrences have taken place. There is also a risk that the engine of the car will explode if the engine is left running for a long time.

There is a Law of the Torah which states that if a piece of wood or metal is burning on the Sabbath in a public place and could be a danger to the lives of people passing by, the flames should be extinguished. The Rambam is of the opinion that a burning piece of wood in such an instance should not be extinguished on the Sabbath but left to burn itself out. However, it is generally agreed that burning metal should be extinguished. The Jerusalem Talmud states that the burning metal should not be extinguished by pouring water over it. A car engine, however, is turned off simply by disconnecting an electrical current. No water is poured on it, which is an added reason for allowing the engine to be turned off.

We may conclude that if the car engine is not turned off, it would be more difficult to find volunteers who would transport emergency cases on the Sabbath in the future, and there is a real danger that the brakes will be damaged and the car will move on its own, or even explode.

I conclude, therefore, that in such a case it is permissible to turn off the engine. Nevertheless, permission should be obtained from the local Rabbi before this is done.

The Gynaecological Examination

HaRav Shmuel HaLevi Wosner,
Rav of Yeshivat Zichron Meir, Bnei Brak

Excerpts from an article in "Pathways in Medicine" 1 (Adar 5739 — March 1979).

Summary: Rabbi Wosner warns Jewish women not to make a habit of having gynaecological examinations, except for those which are definitely necessary.

I have heard that there are Jewish women who frequently and sometimes unnecessarily request gynaecological examinations. I have also heard of cases where gynaecological examinations are carried out very early in pregnancy, without good reason, and of cases where non-religious doctors sometimes carry out such examinations in an immodest manner and in a fashion contrary to the rulings of the Torah. Many great Rabbis have already condemned these practices.

I have discussed elsewhere the practice of newly married couples who visit their gynaecologist in the earliest days of marriage if the wife has not become pregnant. The doctor performs many and varied tests on the wife, and often also asks for specimens of semen from the husband. This practice has no foundation in the Torah. The couple are still young, and there is no need for such tests. The couple carrying out these tests unnecessarily are in fact infringing many precepts of the Torah.

This also applies to many unnecessary visits to the gynaecologist during pregnancy. Such visits break down the barriers of modesty laid down in the Torah. Because I have heard of many such cases, there is no doubt in my mind that this is a matter which should be openly discussed, so that those who do not fully understand the situation, and carry out such practices, can be warned.

In this connection, it is sometimes maintained that such examinations are permissible if the husband is in the same city, as is discussed in Tractate *Kiddushin* 81. I have discussed elsewhere the contention that if a wife speaks to her husband on the telephone just before the examination, perhaps the examination is fully permissible, since it then falls into the category of "the husband being in the same town." I have pointed out that this is not an adequate reason for allowing such examinations. One of the reasons for giving permission if the husband is in the town is that he can come to see his wife at any moment and without warning, but nowadays, in great cities like London, New York and many others, a mere telephone conversation with a husband does not establish that he can suddenly, without warning, come to see his wife. Even though he may be in "the same town," the town is so vast that it may be very difficult for him to appear immediately, without warning. In any case, many great Rabbis insist that we follow the view of Rashi: permission granted on the basis that the husband is in the town is granted only after the fact, but initially his presence in town cannot be used as a reason for granting permission.

I have also heard people maintain that the law prohibiting such examinations only applies to situations where there are no other persons, or very few persons, present, but that if the examination is carried out in a public place where many people may come and go, it is permissible. In support of this contention these persons quote the Rema in *Shulchan Aruch, Even HaEzer* 21. The Rema states that it is permitted to bathe in a public bathhouse when female attendants are present. However, the Bach and other great Rabbis maintain that a God-fearing person should not take advantage of this ruling. In any case, the discussion in the *Shulchan Aruch* refers to cases of normal modesty. In the case of a gynaecological examination, there could be actual contact by the doctor with the female organs. Even though we claim that this is a purely "professional" examination by the doctor, in fact it is a far more serious situation, and in certain circumstances, it may well be that this part of the examination should be forbidden, even if the rest of the examination is permissible. Clearly, the doctor's consulting room is not a public place where many people are passing.

In any case, many doctors of our generation are on a lower spiritual level than the "female attendants" in the bathhouse of former days, for how could the great Rabbis even consider allowing persons to bathe in a bath house where female attendants are present, were it not for the fact that these female attendants were on a high spiritual level, completely beyond suspicion of any evil actions. Surely many doctors nowadays are not on such a spiritual level, unless they are known to be religious and observant.

I wish to make it clear that I had not in any way intended to forbid women from visiting gynaecologists if there is a real need for it, or even if there is the slightest doubt that there may be some danger that necessitates an examination. No Rabbi has the power to forbid such visits. My intention is to warn Jewish ladies to be particularly careful in this matter, and remind them that they should not make any unnecessary visits to the gynaecologist, particularly during the early days of pregnancy or the early days of marriage. Many people do make such unnecessary visits, and they should be warned not to do this, especially in offices which are not strictly private and are situated in immodest surroundings.

Below is a list of various laws and recommendations applicable to visits to the gynaecologist.

1. One should not make a habit of making many visits to the gynaecologist — only when it is absolutely necessary; such visits involve the risk of contravening the laws of modesty as laid down in the Torah.

2. Wherever possible, a female gynaecologist should be consulted.

3. If a particular male doctor happens to be more expert than a female doctor, a visit to the male doctor is preferable, and it cannot be forbidden in any way.

4. If a doctor is known to have behaved immodestly in the past, he should not be visited under any circumstances.

5. One should only visit the gynaecologist by appointment, and at a time when many other patients are also there. At such times, there is less risk of immodesty.

6. One should not visit the gynaecologist alone, but be accompanied by a trusted female companion.

7. In my opinion, it is not advisable for husbands to go with their wives to gynaecological examinations or sit in the waiting room with many women patients.

8. Even though one cannot make a firm ruling on this point, it is preferable, if possible, not to shut the door of the consulting room during the examination. Certainly the door should not be locked.

9. Jewish women should be warned not to follow the advice

of nonreligious gynaecologists concerning contraceptive practices. In all such cases, the advice of a learned Rabbi should be taken first.

10. One should not engage in long conversations with the gynaecologist, but only discuss matters connected with the examination.

Inducing Birth for the Sake of Convenience

HaRav Menashe Klein,
Chief Dayan and Rosh Yeshiva,
Yeshivas Beis Shearim Ungvar, New York

Excerpts from an article in "Pathways in Medicine" 3 - 4 (Av 5740 — July 1980).

Summary: Rabbi Klein shows that it is strictly forbidden to induce a birth by injection or operation when there is no danger to the life of the mother or the child.

Question

The question refers to a normal pregnancy, already in its ninth month, where there is no emergency situation. In such a case, is the doctor permitted to bring on the birth — either by injection or operation — at a time convenient to the parents and the doctor? This procedure ensures that the mother does not have to be rushed unexpectedly to hospital in the middle of the night or on the Sabbath; it helps the father, who otherwise may not be at home when labor begins; and it is convenient for the doctor, who may not be immediately available at the time the pregnancy completes its full course. Such a procedure would avoid undue haste and enable the birth to take place at a time when everything necessary has been prepared.

Answer

It is a clear principle of the Torah that a person is normally forbidden to put himself into a dangerous situation. One reason for this principle is that to do so is a form of ingratitude to the Creator, Who wishes to do good to human beings. Instead of being grateful, the human being unnecessarily endangers his life, revealing a lack of appreciation for the great goodness of Hashem.

It is also clear that birth is a time of danger for mother and infant. The Talmud refers to the fact that during birth an accusing Angel may attempt to emphasise the shortcomings and wrongdoings of the mother. The accusing Angel is especially active in time of danger, and at such times, people sometimes require miracles to save them. The Abarbanel states that a mother who has just given birth is instructed to bring a special offering to the Temple as a sign of gratitude to Hashem for bringing her safely out of the danger through which she has just passed. In addition, we are allowed to violate the Sabbath in order to assist a mother who is giving birth. And for three days after birth, she is still regarded as an ill person for whom the Sabbath may be violated. Thus it is clear that a normal birth is regarded by the Torah as a time of danger.

It is all the more dangerous to bring birth on before its time. The Torah tells us that at the natural time for a birth, Hashem shows special kindness and prepares the mother so the birth will be easy. If we select our own time for the birth, it may well be that this special kindness will be affected.

There is another danger which must be considered. If an injection is used to bring on the birth, it is known that it might not act with sufficient strength, and this may sometimes injure the mother. Such things can also happen with a birth which occurs at the natural time, but we have a principle: we ourselves should not bring danger nearer. If the birth is performed through an operation, it is even more dangerous. It is forbidden to undergo any such serious operation if it is not absolutely necessary.

Such a procedure can also endanger the infant, who is very weak in any case. In His goodness, Hashem normally allots nine months for the infant to gain strength and develop. The Talmud tells us that we are unable to be sure that the fetus has reached the age of nine months, as we do not know the exact date when the development of the fetus began. When a pregnancy is induced, a mistake may be made, and the fetus may be only eight months old, which can be dangerous to the infant, even if it is kept in an incubator after birth. I know of a case where the wife of one of my students was given an injection in order to bring on birth on the assumption that the fetus was already nine months old. A mistake was made, and a premature birth took place. The newborn infant had to be kept in an incubator for six weeks, and the child was always smaller than usual for his age and generally weaker. I have also heard of a tragic case where the infant died as the result of an induced premature birth.

There is a more mystical and spiritual factor which deserves consideration in this context. The Talmud tells us that when a child is conceived, an angel brings the seed before Hashem, Who decides whether the infant is to be rich or poor and how his life will proceed. The question of whether he will be righteous or wicked is not decided, as this depends on free will. The *Zohar* tells us that just before a child is born, Hashem judges him and determines whether he is fit to be born. We believe that the actual date of birth can have some influence on thse deliberations. If we change the date of birth that was determined in

Heaven, it may well have a harmful influence on the fate of the infant.

Again, according to Jewish tradition, as the Talmud explains, the best time of a person's life is the time he spends in the womb. The Talmud says that during these nine months, an angel teaches the unborn infant the secrets of the whole Torah, and a light shines that enables the infant to see from one end of the world to the other. All this is forgotten and wiped out at the moment of birth. It may be that if we shorten the time in the womb, we may be shortening the infant's spiritual development.

I would like to add that I have even heard of cases where the birth was induced on a Sunday, because the parents wished to have the circumcision on the following Sunday so that more guests would be able to attend. From all we have said, it is clear that such actions are completely forbidden by the Torah.

In this connection, I have also been asked if it is permissible to pray that a mother give birth speedily and without delay in cases where the pregnancy is difficult. This is in no way forbidden, and it is indeed praiseworthy.

Religious parents should be advised that the procedures discussed above are to be condemned. If a doctor advises such a procedure, his advice should not be followed.

I wish to make it clear that if there is any danger to the health of the mother or the infant, and for this reason the doctor advises such a procedure, it would be a grave sin not to follow the advice of the doctor. Where there is a risk to life, the doctor's advice must always be followed. The cases discussed above are all situations where there is no danger to life and no serious reason to induce labour.

Taking Medicine on the Sabbath

HaRav Chayim David Leifer,
Rav, Sanz Synagogue of Haifa;
Rabbinical Committee of Laniado Hospital

Excerpts from an article in "Pathways in Medicine" 7(Elul 5745-September 1985).

Summary: Rabbi Leifer discusses a commonly held tradition that one may take medicine on the Sabbath if he is merely feeling a little "indisposed," and is not actually ill, provided that one has already been taking the medicine for one or two days before the Sabbath. He quotes Talmudic sources in support of his view that this is an incorrect tradition, and concludes that one should *not* take medicine on the Sabbath if he is merely feeling "indisposed," but only if he could *suffer* from illness if he does not take it on the Sabbath.

There is a commonly held tradition, handed down among the Jewish people, that if a sick person has begun a course of medicine before the Sabbath, and the doctor has prescribed that the medicine be taken for a number of days, which would include the Sabbath, he is permitted to take the medicine on the Sabbath. This tradition is mentioned in *Sefer HaChayim* (chap. 6, par. 328). It seems to me that perhaps this tradition may have arisen from the Talmud (*Shabbos* 140) in the section dealing with *asafoetida*, a plant which was used as a medicine, and is referred to in the Talmud by its Aramaic name, *hiltit*. The *Shulchan Aruch, Orach Chayim* 321:18, is based on this section of the Talmud.

I have always found this tradition very difficult to understand. It's clear that this section of the Talmud refers to a patient who, if he does not continue to take medicine on the Sabbath, is putting himself in *danger*. This is also stated in the *Shulchan Aruch*. From this we learn that the permission granted for the patient to continue to take the medicine on the Sabbath is conditional on the fact that if he does not take it, *he will be putting himself in danger*. If there is no danger from his not taking the medicine for one day, he is *forbidden* to continue taking the medicine on the Sabbath!

In *Sefer HaChayim* quoted above, the question of whether or not the patient would put himself in danger by stopping the medicine on the Sabbath is not referred to at all. This calls for clarification. I found that this difficulty is actually mentioned in *Orchos HaChayim* 328:37, in the name of the Marhasham. It is also raised in *Da'as Torah* 328:37.

In *Shemiras Shabbos KeHilchasah* 21:10, one can apparently find some support for the tradition mentioned above. The author cites the commentary of the Ran on Tractate *Shabbos*: "There are some who maintain that in this instance the word 'danger' does not refer to actual danger, but merely to someone who is *suffering* from his illness, as in the other case we discussed, and both these cases refer to a person who is ill, but not desperately ill."

It would seem that the author of *Shemiras Shabbos KeHilchasah* is saying as follows: Because the Ran states that the case referred to is not one of actual danger — the patient is only *suffering* from his illness — it follows that a patient may continue to take the medicine on the Sabbath even if he is only *suffering* as a result of his illness. According to the Ran, therefore, as quoted in *Shemiras Shabbos KeHilchasah,* the tradition that one may continue to take medicine if one has begun before the Sabbath can refer to a case where one would *suffer* if he stopped taking the medicine on the Sabbath.

Our original difficulty remains. The Ran states that "both cases refer to a person who is ill, but not dangerously ill." From this it follows that the Talmud is considering a case where the patient is ill, but not dangerously ill — that is, he would *suffer* if did not take the medicine on the Sabbath, and, therefore, is permitted to continue to take it on the Sabbath. However, according to the *Sefer HaChayim* quoted above, the tradition that we are discussing states that a person can continue to take the medicine on the Sabbath even if he is feeling *"indisposed,"* and not necessarily *"suffering."*

Later I found, in the second edition of *Shemiras Shabbos KeHilchasah* 34:76, that the author appears to have reconsidered the matter; he does not seem to accept the view of the *Sefer HaChayim.* The author states: "The Gaon Rabbi S. Z. Auerbach told me that this case refers to a patient who will become ill if he does not continue to take the medicine on the Sabbath, but not to a patient who will merely be indisposed. He emphasises that the words of the Ran refer only to a case where a person is *suffering* from 'an illness which is not dangerous,' and not to a mere 'indisposition.' "

From this discussion it is clear that one cannot take medicine merely because he feels indisposed. All the sources quoted above refers only to a person who would be ill if he did not take the medicine on the Sabbath and not if the person was merely indisposed.

This view can also be learned from a close examination of a section of Tractate *Avodah Zarah* 28. There Rav Eliezer asks if the toothache he is suffering from can be considered an internal illness. The Talmud answers by citing the case of Rabbi Yochanan, who was suffering from a toothache. Thursday had passed, and the Sabbath was approaching. Rabbi Yochanan asked: "What can I do about this tomorrow?" The Talmud seeks to bring a proof from Rabbi Yohanan's question that the toothache was considered to be "internal," and therefore a more serious illness. Rashi explains that since he was seeking to take medicine for his illness on the Sabbath, it follows that his toothache must have been considered to be an internal, and therefore a more serious, illness, otherwise he would not have even asked the question.

Now, if one who began taking medicine before the Sabbath may continue taking it on the Sabbath even if the illness was merely an "indisposition," then why would Rabbi Yohanan even trouble himself to ask the question: "What can I do about this tomorrow?" He clearly had been taking the medicine before the Sabbath (The Talmud states: "Thursday had passed, and the Sabbath was approaching"), and, therefore, it would have been permissible for him to take the medicine on the Sabbath, even if his toothache were not serious.

Even though I feel that the commonly held tradition we have discussed should not be followed, I have still tried to find some support for it; although the Jewish people are not prophets, they are descended from prophets, and one must seriously consider a widely-held tradition. In actual practice, however, I am of the opinion that we must follow the sources quoted from the Talmud and the opinions of the great Rabbis, which are contrary to that tradition.

Conclusion

On considering all these sources, I have come to the conclusion that one should *not* take medicine on the Sabbath if one is merely "indisposed," even if he has been taking the medicine for several days before the Sabbath, but only *if he would actually suffer* if he did not take it.

Heart Transplants

HaRav Shmuel HaLevi Wosner,
Rav of Yeshivat Zichron Meir,
Bnei Brak

Excerpts from an article in "Pathways in Medicine" 8 (Kislev 5747 — January 1987).

Summary: Rabbi Wosner brings proofs from the Torah that a patient may not be declared dead until his heart has stopped beating. He demonstrates that even those Rabbis in the Talmud who maintain that one need only examine the patient for signs of breathing from the nostrils when ascertaining death, actually refer to special cases, and in fact they agree that the true criterion for the declaration of death is whether or not the heart is still beating. If a patient's heart is still beating, the patient is alive; removal of his heart for the purpose of a transplant operation *does in fact cause that patient's death,* and is therefore forbidden according to Jewish law.

Just before Sabbath, I received a letter in which the problem of heart transplants was mentioned. This problem has been discussed a great deal lately, and many scholarly Rabbis have considered the matter according to the rulings of the Torah. All of them raise very serious doubts about this procedure. Many doctors, some of whom are not overly concerned about the "principles of humanity," have also stated opinions, on one side or the other. I have, therefore, decided to set down some of the basic opinions stated by our learned Rabbis and by the great Rabbinical scholars of the previous generations. (See *Chacham Zvi, no. 77; Chasam Sofer, Yoreh De'ah,* no. 338; *Darkei Chayim, Even HaEzer* vol. 2; *Minchas Yitzchak,* vol. 5, no. 70.)

A. The basic question which must be considered is whether death is to be determined by cessation of life in the heart or cessation of life in the brain as indicated by the end of breathing. In other words, do we confirm that the heart has stopped beating before we declare that patient dead, or do we declare the patient dead when his breathing has ended — apparent death of the brain — *even though his heart may still be beating*!

In Tractate *Yoma* 85, the following question is asked: how should a suspected dead person be examined? One answer is that he should be examined from his head to his nostrils, in which case it would appear that there is no need to examine the heart. Another answer is that he need only be examined from his feet up to and including his heart.

The first opinion appears to be saying that when the question arises, at what point is there no longer an obligation to strive to save a person's life? the final decision as to whether or not a person is still alive must depend on whether or not breath is still passing through his nostrils.

The following verse is quoted in support of this view: "All who have breath of life in their nostrils" (Bereshis 7:22).

However, the second opinion, which states that the examination should be made from the feet upwards, clearly believes that if the heart has stopped functioning, no further examination is necessary; life dependes on the continued function of the heart. (The view of modern science would appear to follow the first opinion.)

However, this is not the correct explanation of the first

of the Chacham Zvi (no. 77) and the Chasam Sofer (*Yoreh De'ah*, no. 338), who maintain that according to both opinions *the beating of the heart is the decisive factor*, and a patient cannot be considered dead until his heart has stopped beating, even if he has stopped breathing. The Chacham Zvi emphasises that this view is supported by many indisputable arguments from other learned Rabbis, the Zohar, and the writings of Saadiah Gaon. (See Responsa, *Yoreh De'ah*, no. 116.) Therefore, *as long as the heart is still functioning, the patient must be considered still alive*, and it is forbidden to do anything which may cause him to die or hasten his death, even if his breathing has stopped. The view of the Chacham Zvi is accepted by Jewish law, and in this important matter erroneous and irrelevant arguments based only on scientific opinions must not be taken into consideration. The Chasam Sofer states clearly that if his heart is still beating, even though there is no sign of breathing, the patient must still be regarded as alive. However, if the patient lies cold and lifeless, and there is no heartbeat, we must declare the patient dead. This is, in fact, the condition stated by the Torah for determining death after the death sentence has been carried out on a criminal.

False argument brought forward by a scientist

Under no circumstances can we accept the words written by a certain scientist, that the Rabbis of former generations were in general not correct in their opinions, as their opinions were not based on fact. This scientist concludes that the Rabbis are not correct when they say that the beating of the heart determines life or death; he claims that death can be determined by the death of the brain, in accord with the discoveries of science. Such a statement must be regarded as erroneous and harmful.

In the matter which we are considering, not one Rabbi differs with the views stated by the Chacham Zvi and the Chasam Sofer — life is to be determined by the continued functioning of the heart — and this view is based on rulings and traditions handed down from the earliest days, when the Torah was revealed to the Jewish people. We must follow only the opinions stated by our Rabbis and cannot accept opinions which doctors attempt to force on us. Furthermore, we maintain that the "facts" which the doctors place before us are not "facts" at all, and cannot in any way overrule our traditional law, which states that as long as the heart is alive, the patient is still alive, even if the brain has ceased to function and breathing has stopped. It is almost a certainty that, at some time in the future, scientists will suddenly discover and announce to the world that if the patient's heart is still functioning, especially without assistance from a life-support machine, the roots of the brain have not completely died, and that there is a connection, albeit hidden, between the living heart and the brain, and the patient is therefore not dead!

B. We must still explain the view quoted earlier, that in order to determine whether a patient is dead, one should examine him from the head downwards, only until the nostrils. It does appear at first sight that, according to this view, it is sufficient to check breathing through the nostrils, and not the heart, when determining death. Clearly this is not the true explanation of the view held by this group of Rabbis. The Rabbis here are referring to a particular case: The person being examined has had a fall, and his brain has been damaged to such an extent that it can be said to have become separated completely from the body. In such a case, there is no doubt that the person is dead; it is as if his head had been cut off from his body! These Rabbis wish to explain to us that *in this particular case,* even if the body is still showing signs of movement, such movement is of no significance because the head is so badly damaged that it can be regarded as if it had been completely severed from the body. (See *Ohalos*, chap. 1 and Rambam at the end of the first chapter of *Hilchos Tumas Meis* and the end of the fourth chapter of *Hilchos She'ar Avos HaTumah*.)

In fact, it is clear that the Rabbis who tell us to examine the patient from the head downwards until the nostrils intend to include an examination of the sides of the head and the sides of the neck, where one can see if there is any sign of the pulse from the beating of the heart. If *no* breath is coming from the nostrils and there are no signs of a pulse at the sides of the head and neck, we are permitted to declare that the patient is dead. But if there *are* signs of a pulse, the patient cannot be declared dead!

One could still raise the following question: Even if there are no signs of breath in the nostrils and no pulse in the neck or on the sides of the head, is there still a possibility, however remote, that the heart may still be beating without enough strength to cause movement in the nostrils or on the sides of the neck or head? Does this not indicate that, according to this view, the condition of the heart need not be considered at all?

Again, this would not be a correct explanation of this view. The situation in Tractate *Yoma* is a special case — a person fell from a height, say, in a landslide, and was covered up by earth. When some of the earth was removed, and the upper part of his body uncovered, from the head until the nostrils, there were no signs of life, either on the sides of the head or on the neck, and no signs of pulse or breath in the nostrils. Then the halachic ruling is that we can declare the person dead. We do not have to suspect that there is, in spite of all the signs of death, some sign of life in the heart. It is clear that this is a unique ruling and in all other cases the heart must be examined before declaring death. This special case is not comparable to a heart transplant operation, where it is *perfectly clear* that the heart *is* still alive, and *must*, in fact, still be beating when the transplant operation is being performed! We must, therefore, conclude that according to Jewish Law, if the heart is still beating, the patient is still alive. It is completely forbidden to remove a living heart from a patient in order to transfer it to another patient. By doing so we are, in fact, killing the first patient. Heart transplant operations must be regarded as strictly forbidden according to the Torah; they involve the removal of a living heart from a patient who, from the point of view of Jewish Law, is "alive" while his heart is being removed in order to transplant it into another patient.

Furthermore, it is well known that the heart of a patient who appears to be dying can continue to beat for a considerable time.

In addition to the fact that the performance of a heart transplant will certainly cause the death of the donor, there is another aspect of this matter which gives me concern. I doubt that this form of treatment is permitted at all according to the rulings of the Torah. As Rabbeinu Bachya states in his commentary on *parashas Mishpatim*, a doctor is permitted to heal according to the ruling of the Bible, which states, "Thou shalt surely heal." However, there is an opinion that this permission to heal refers only to "external" treatment, not to the treatment of internal organs. Although this view has not been accepted as halachically binding by later generations, there must be some basis for it.

Furthermore, a heart transplant works against the very basis of the creation of the human being — it makes a fundamental change in the Divine plan of Creation. The transfer of a vital organ from one person to another changes the plan laid down by the Creator when He created the two persons. One may well ask who gave the doctors the permission and the authority to perform such actions? This objection is in addition to the point already made: that the greatest Torah scholars have ruled that such operations, without doubt, fall within the definition of the killing of a human being.

There is another important point to bear in mind. I have been advised by medical specialists that it is extremely likely that the glucose injection usually administered to a heart or liver donor before his death, whose purpose is to preserve the freshness of the organ to be transplanted, can actually hasten the donor's death! How can we put complete trust in what the doctors and hospital staff do at such a moment of crisis?

Conclusion

We must state that the views of our great Torah scholars, which forbid such operations according to the ruling of the Torah, must be accepted without any hesitation or doubt.

We must trust that the Almighty in His great mercy will ensure that the blood of the innocent is not shed, and let us all strive to do what is right in the eyes of the Lord!

Abortion for an Expectant Mother with German Measles

HaRav Meir Bransdorfer,
Dayan, Rabbinical Court of Jerusalem

Excerpts from an article in "Pathways in Medicine" 2 (Elul 5739 — September 1979).

Summary: Rabbi Bransdorfer was asked if an abortion could be performed to terminate a pregnancy in a case where the mother had contracted German measles. He concludes that such an abortion is strictly forbidden by Jewish Law, except where there is definite medical evidence that the continuation of the pregnancy will endanger the life of the mother.

Question

The question concerns a mother who, unfortunately, contracted German measles at the beginning of her pregnancy. The doctors decided there was a risk that the newborn would be deficient in some of its limbs or have an impaired intelligence. They recommended that an abortion be performed. They stated that this would avoid the birth of a human being who would suffer pain and sorrow and cause suffering to the parents. In addition, the parents would be saved the trouble and effort required to bring up such an infant. The question asked was: Is it permissible, according to Jewish Law, to accept the advice of the doctors and allow the abortion to be performed?

Answer

It is clear beyond any doubt that in Jewish Law, under normal circumstances, an abortion is completely forbidden. It is regarded as murder. There is an opinion in Tractate *Sanhedrin* 57 that a non-Jew can be sentenced to death if he intentionally causes the death of a fetus in the womb while a Jew cannot be put to death for such a crime. While there is considerable discussion among the Rabbis concerning this opinion, it is nevertheless clear that even if a Jew should not be put to death for killing a fetus in the womb, he is forbidden to carry out such an action by Biblical decree, which classifies such an action as a form of murder.

In what circumstances is it permissible to abort according to Jewish Law?

Jewish Law does state that a fetus which is likely to cause the death of the mother can be aborted. The permission to abort in such a case is based on the following arguments.

Our Rabbis state that one should not have mercy on a person who wishes to kill him. It is permitted to kill such a person in self-defence. From this principle, the Rabbis also learn that if a fetus in the womb is in such a condition that the mother would not be able to give birth normally, and may die as a result, it is permitted to operate on the fetus in the womb, with drugs or surgery, since the unborn infant can be regarded as being in the same category as a person who wishes to kill another person, and can, therefore, if necessary, be killed first. The Torah lays down a condition, however: if most of the head has already been born, then this should not be done; the baby is to be regarded as if already born. This view — that a fetus which is a danger to the life of the mother may be killed — conforms with the opinion of some of the Rabbis, who argue that until it is born, it is not to be regarded as a complete living soul.

There are other Rabbis who question the permission to abort. These Rabbis ask how a fetus which can cause the death of the mother can be killed on the grounds that it is comparable to a murderer pursuing a person with the intention of killing him. They claim that such a fetus cannot be regarded as being in the same category as a "pursuing murderer." This situation is clearly a case of an illness which has been brought on the mother and child by Heavenly Decree. It cannot be said to have arisen through the wicked intention of the unborn child, as is the case with a murderer, who should be killed before he can kill.

The Rabbis who do believe that such a fetus should be aborted, answer by saying that until it is born, it is not to be regarded as a complete soul. Therefore, killing such a fetus in the womb is not to be regarded as murder, but only a kind of derivative of murder. In addition, even though it cannot be classed as a "pursuing murderer," nevertheless, since it is the actual cause of the possible death of the mother, it can be regarded as "related to a murderer." Therefore, the Torah tells us that in such a case it is permitted to operate on the unborn child if it is certain that the mother's life would be endangered during birth.

A fetus may be aborted if it is a danger to the life of the mother, but if the continuance of the pregnancy will not endanger the life of the mother in any way, an abortion is strictly forbidden

It is clear from all this discussion, that, according to Jewish Law, the only possible rationale for giving permission to abort a fetus is that it is comparable to a "pursuing murderer," in which case it must be killed before it can cause the death of the mother. However, if the pregnancy will in no way risk the mother's life, *it is clear that it is strictly forbidden to abort.*

The fetus whose mother has contracted German measles will not, as a rule, endanger the mother's life if the pregnancy is allowed to continue

In the case in question concerning the mother who had contracted German measles, the fetus was clearly not a cause of danger to the mother at all. Thus, even if the fetus is not yet forty days old, when, according to some opinions, it is not yet formed into a fetus, it would still be strictly forbidden to abort it, since it did not constitute a danger to the life of the mother.

We may violate the Sabbath or the Day of Atonement in order to save an unborn child

Indeed, our Rabbis tell us that we may even violate the Sabbath in order to save the life of an unborn child; one Sabbath may be violated to ensure that the newborn baby will, hopefully, observe many Sabbaths in the future. They add that one must not even stand by and do nothing if the unborn child is sick, but every effort must be made to save its life. If we may even violate the Sabbath to save the life of an unborn child, how much more so would it be completely forbidden to kill the fetus while it is in the womb. In addition, the Torah tells us that if the unborn child is sick, the mother is permitted to eat on the Day of Atonement if it will save the unborn baby's life. It is therefore quite clear that whenever there is no danger to life, it is forbidden.

Conclusion: No abortion should be carried out in the case of a mother who has contracted German measles, unless there is a definite medical opinion that continuing the pregnancy would endanger the mother's life.

The Test-Tube Baby and the "Recipient Mother"

HaRav Moshe Sternbuch,
Rosh Yeshiva, Yeshivat Rosh Ha'ayin

Excepts from an article in "Pathways in Medicine" 8 (Kislev 5747 — January 1987).

Summary: Rabbi Sternbuch discusses the problems connected with the test-tube baby and the "recipient mother." He comes to the conclusion that the test-tube baby procedure is not permissible in Jewish Law. The "recipient mother" procedure also opens the door to many dangerous and complicated situations, for example, when the donor is found to be a non-Jewish woman, while the mother who gave birth is Jewish.

I would like to refer to a question which was put to me in Johannesburg. A lady whose fallopian tubes were obstructed had been advised by her doctors that there was no possibility she could have a normal pregnancy. Her doctors recommended a test-tube pregnancy, a procedure that had been available for the past ten years. The principle of this method of pregnancy is that the female eggs are removed and joined with sperm which has been taken from the husband. These are then placed in a sterile test-tube, in which the egg is fertilised. It is then planted into the mother's womb, where the fetus grows normally until birth. The lady advised me that she and her husband were very distressed over the fact that they had been unable to have children, and her husband had even considered divorce. She was indeed depressed over her situation, and she had come to ask me if, according to Jewish Law, she was permitted to go through the test-tube baby procedure.

There is no question of abortion in the test-tube baby procedure

I have heard it stated that the test-tube baby procedure should be forbidden because it could result in an abortion which would be considered to be murder according to Jewish law. Those who forbid the procedure for this reason maintain that after the female eggs and male sperm have already been fertilised in the test tube, the doctors often destroy the contents of the tube and perform the procedure over and over again, until they find that the fertilisation has been the best possible according to their standards. According to those who wish to forbid the procedure for this reason, destruction of the material in the test tube is in fact a form of abortion, which should be forbidden.

I do not agree with this line of argument. It appears to me that an abortion can only take place when the fetus is already in the mother's womb. In this case, the developing fetus is still not in the mother's womb when it is destroyed. Another procedure still has to be followed to plant the embryo in the womb. It appears quite clearly to me that the destruction of the material in the test tube can in no way be considered to be a case of abortion, or murder, of an embryo.

In the test-tube baby procedure, according to Jewish law, the husband cannot be considered to be the natural father

In Jewish Law, a father can only be considered the "natural" father of an infant when the infant has been conceived through normal marital relations between husband and wife. One must conclude that in the case of the test-tube baby procedure, where there are no normal marital relations, the husband cannot be considered the natural father. Moreover, the emission of sperm by the husband would not be permissible in Jewish Law, because sperm must only be emitted in order to conceive directly. While there are some great Rabbis who do permit artificial fertilisation in cases of great need, they, in fact, only permit such a procedure when male sperm is inserted directly into the mother's womb. In the case of a test-tube baby, there is an intermediary which actually effects the growth of the embryo — the test-tube — and the procedure is even further removed from a normal marital relationship.

We conclude that according to the opinion of all the Rabbis, when the egg is fertilised in a test-tube, the husband cannot be considered the natural father of the newborn infant, and the emission of sperm by the father in order to carry out such a procedure would not be permissible.

An additional reason to forbid the test-tube procedure

There is another reason to forbid this procedure. It may well be that if we allow this procedure we would open the door to the disintegration of the basis of Jewish family life, genealogy and descent. How could we be sure that no errors take place? Perhaps the father's sperm will accidentally be exchanged for the sperm of another man? A brother may become the father of his sister's baby through an error! We must always remember that the holiness of the Jewish nation is based on the preservation of our "family tree" or, as the Torah says: "Families are established through their fathers." How can we be sure that no mistakes are made, even if we are talking about very conscientious and reliable doctors? Our Rabbis have a duty to guard the sanctity of the Jewish family. I once discussed this point with a doctor in Johannesburg who is an international authority on the subject, and he fully agreed with me that my fears were justified. He even said to me: "The Rabbis should do their job, and we, the doctors should do our job. We should look after the health of the ladies, and you should protect the holiness of the Jewish family."

The Torah tells us the story of Yisro, the father-in-law of Moshe, who was highly praised and honoured for giving Moshe advice which he accepted. He advised Moshe to appoint assistant judges to judge the people, because if Moshe continued to deal with all the people's problems himself, he would surely wear himself out. We may comment that Moshe was possessed of an unusual strength, and Yisro could surely see that he was quite capable of performing the task he had set for himself without any need for assistance. Yisro's greatness lay in the fact that he realised that if Moshe were allowed to continue to judge the people later, weaker judges who followed him would adopt the same method, and as a result the whole observance of Jewish Law could be seriously harmed. Similarly, in our case, even if we are sure that in a particular instance we are dealing with a highly skilled and conscientious doctor who will not make an error, we should remember the lesson of Yisro. If we allow this procedure in a case where the doctors are known to be conscientious, the procedure will become acceptable, and other less conscientious doctors will be allowed to carry it out, with disastrous results for Jewish family sanctity.

Therefore, even though I felt deeply sorry for the distressed couple who came to me with their question, I felt I had to forbid the procedure for the reasons I have stated.

The case of the non-Jewish donor to a Jewish recipient mother

I wish now to consider a case where the female eggs are produced by one woman and transplanted into the womb of another woman. The fetus grows in the second woman's womb, and she gives birth. The question may be asked: who is the true mother according to Jewish Law? Is it the first woman, who produced the female eggs, or the second one, who gave birth to the infant? Perhaps both women should be considered the mothers! We must remember that the procedures we have been discussing are becoming more and more common; thousands of women have already given birth this way. Usually, the doctor carrying out the procedure treats both Jewish and non-Jewish mothers. What would be if the eggs produced by a non-Jewish mother were planted in the womb of a Jewish mother? Would the infant be considered Jewish, or non-Jewish, in which case a conversion ceremony might be necessary? If we say that the actual birth and the period of growth in the womb are the deciding factors, then the infant is Jewish. On the other hand, we could say that there is still an influence from the mother who originally produced the eggs, and the development of the fetus in the womb cannot remove that influence. From this point of view, the infant would be required to undergo a form of conversion immediately after birth in order to be recognised as fully Jewish. This is similar to a case in Tractate *Yevamos* 97, where a non-Jewish pregnant woman decided to convert to Judaism before she gave birth and then gave birth to male twins. The Ramban says that the twins should go through a conversion ceremony before circumcision. If we follow the opinion that the true mother of the child is the mother who gave birth to the child, the infant would be permitted to marry close relatives (e.g., the children) of the first woman who donated her eggs to the mother. One can readily see that the situation could become quite terrifying, since sperm and eggs are sometimes frozen for many years, and even used after their donors are no longer alive. The basis of the sanctity of the Jewish family could be said to be endangered by the use of such procedures.

We recall the Midrash which relates that when the Torah was given to the Jewish people on Mount Sinai, the non-Jewish nations were jealous, and they asked the Almighty why they were also not entitled to receive the Torah. The Midrash states that they were asked to bring forward their "family trees" and show how each family was derived from its father, as the Children of Israel had been able to do. As the non-Jewish nations were unable to do this, they were not entitled to receive the Torah. From this we may learn that the basis of Jewish purity is the purity of the family, and the dangers of the procedures we have been discussing are, therefore, evident.

After due consideration, I have concluded that in the case of the transplanted eggs, the true mother is the mother who gave birth to the child, and there is no connection with the donor who produced the eggs.

However, I have not been able to find this law clearly stated in any work. I therefore feel that if there is any risk at all that the donor of the female egg was not Jewish, the newborn infant should pass through a conversion ceremony.

Is a Particular Doctor Decreed to Cure a Patient?

HaRav Yitzchak Zilberstein,
Av Beit Din, Ramat Elchanan, Bnei Brak;
Rabbinical Committee of Laniado Hospital

Excerpts from an article in "Pathways in Medicine" 2 (Elul 5739—September 1979).

Summary: Rabbi Zilberstein brings illustrations from the Talmud and from actual incidents that have taken place to demonstrate that it is possible that a particular doctor and a particular cure have been assigned to a patient by Heavenly decree.

The Talmud (*Avodah Zarah* 55) states: "When suffering is decreed upon a man, the sufferings have to make an oath in Heaven, that they will only depart from that man on a certain decreed day, at a certain decreed time, through the treatment of a particular person, and through the action of a particular medicine."

At first sight, this statement is difficult to understand. It says that a patient is cured only by means of one particular medicine which has been decreed in Heaven. It also states that only one doctor has the power to use that medicine and cure that patient, the doctor who has been appointed to do so in Heaven! Does this mean that another doctor, however well qualified, will not be able to effect a cure?

We find a similar situation in Tractate *Nedarim* 41. The Talmud speaks of a person who has vowed that he will receive no benefit from a particular person. If the person who made the vow is a doctor, and the other person falls ill, the doctor is allowed to treat that person, in spite of his vow, even if there are other doctors available who are capable of treating him. The Talmud explains its ruling with the phrase: "A man cannot be cured by everyone," suggesting that a particular person — the person who made the vow — may well be the person decreed in Heaven to cure the patient, and he is therefore permitted to break his vow.

Let us look further into the Talmud to find a deeper explanation for these statements, which appear at first sight to be contrary to normal medical experience. In Tractate *Bava Metzia* 110, the following case is quoted: A certain man receives instructions from the owner of a field to sow a field with wheat. The tenant farmer ignores the instructions and sows the field with barley instead of wheat. All the crops in the area are suddenly stricken by a crop disease. The tenant farmer is obliged to compensate the farmer for the loss of his crop. The Talmud asks why the tenant farmer cannot claim that all the crops in the area were stricken by the same disease, and it was not his fault? The answer given is that the owner of the field is entitled to say to the tenant farmer that if he had followed his instructions, and sowed wheat and not barley, the crop might not have been affected by the disease. The Talmud quotes a passage from Iyov which suggests that there are people who can give instructions, and what they desire is granted to them exactly according to their instructions.

At first glance, this story is very difficult to understand. It seems to suggest that the owner of the field had the power to work miracles and overrule the forces of nature. However, the Talmud intends to teach us a deep lesson, which is applicable to the questions we raised at the beginning of this article. One should never underestimate the spiritual power of an individual Jew! Is it not possible that at one time the owner of the field had performed an outstandingly good deed, and, as a result, it was decreed in Heaven that his wishes and desires should be fulfiled, and if the tenant farmer had followed his instructions and sowed the crop the owner told him to sow, the crop would, indeed, not have been stricken? As the Klausenberger Rebbe, *ztz"l*, once explained, righteous people, who go beyond the limits of human nature to perform good deeds, are rewarded by the Almighty; He is willing to overrule the laws of nature to reward them.

We are reminded of the story of Gideon. He once saw his father ploughing one of his fields. Suddenly, the Midianites, who were besieging the area, began to shoot hundreds of arrows in the direction of the field. The Bible relates that Gideon told his father to return home. The field had to be ploughed, and he wished to give honour to his father, so he went into the field and ploughed it under fire of the Midianite arrows. The Bible tells us that because he was not afraid to risk such danger in order to honour his father, he was granted a reward — he was chosen to lead the victorious armies of Israel in the forthcoming battle!

Thus it may well be, that because of certain good deeds that a doctor performed, he has been chosen in Heaven to effect the cure and receive reward for doing so, and it would be against the wishes of Heaven if another, "unworthy" doctor, was called upon to perform this task. It may well be that there is another doctor in the vicinity, one who has done evil deeds, and there is a divine decree that the good doctor should be called to heal the patient instead of the other doctor, who is not entitled to take credit for the cure.

A story is told about the late Rav Yitzchak Elchonon, the famous Rav of Kovno, author of *Be'er Yitzchak*. A wealthy man approached him and offered to cover the expenses of publishing his book. The Rav surprised his disciples by refusing to accept financial assistance from the wealthy man. The donor tried to persuade him. He said that he had always been upright in business, and there was no reason for the Rav to refuse to accept his money. When the man pressed hard, the Rav cried out, "No! No! I am unable to accept this money!"

After the wealthy man left the Rav's room, his students asked him to explain his action. He calmly told them that as soon as the wealthy man entered his room the Rav recognised him, although the man did not recognise him. As a child, Rav Yitzchak Elchonon had been a penniless orphan. On one occasion his shoes needed repair, and he had no money to repair them. He went to this very same wealthy man and begged him for a donation so that he could repair his shoes. The man harshly refused. Rav Yitzchak Elchonon then asked if the wealthy man could lend him the money, which he would pay back when he was an adult. Again the wealthy man refused and drove him from his door. The Rav went on to explain: "Now that I am the Rav of Kovno, he wants to buy a share in my learning. If he had given me the money to repair my shoes then, I might have been able to write more holy books. This man has no right to receive a portion of my holy writings!"

In our case, is it not possible that a doctor who has done evil things, say, driven away a poor orphan from his door, has not been granted in Heaven the right to cure the patient, while another doctor, who has done good deeds, is the one who must administer the medicine and cure the patient — by Heavenly decree?

There is another point to be considered. A doctor who is a good person and who has done many good deeds in the past may well be able to give such powerful spiritual encouragement to the patient that this in itself will be sufficient to effect the cure. The work *Yalkut Me'am Lo'ez* talks about a man who is suffering financial stress and sees that his wife is praying for him. This alone can bring him such joy and be such a source of encouragement, that it can change his whole life and relieve him of his financial difficulties.

I would like to conclude this article with an incident that was related to me by a great Rabbi. It clearly illustrates the point I have been emphasising.

The Rabbi told me that he had once suffered a severe heart attack and been rushed to hospital. A doctor approached him and asked if he was the Rabbi whom he had once heard deliver a lecture on a certain subject in the Talmud. When he received a positive answer, the doctor said he was delighted to have been given the opportunity to treat the Rabbi, as he would be able to clarify certain difficult points that he had not fully understood in the lecture. The Rabbi confided to me that, at that time, he uttered a prayer of thanks to the Almighty who had put him into the hands of a doctor who knew him and respected him. The doctor examined the Rabbi and said: "Please excuse me if I leave you now. I can see from my examination that you are not seriously ill, and I must attend to some seriously ill patients." Once again the Rabbi thanked the Almighty for the doctor's comforting words. But his happiness changed to fear and distress when a group of nurses suddenly appeared at his bedside and rushed him to the emergency ward, where he was fitted with many tubes and dials. The Rabbi knew then that he was indeed seriously ill. He saw the same doctor again standing by his bed. "Why have you lied to me?" he cried. "You can see how seriously ill I am!" The doctor spoke to him again in comforting tones: "Not at all. You are not seriously ill. It so happens that you are in need of a good rest. Where you were was much too noisy, and there was a spare bed in the emergency ward where it's much quieter. So I gave instructions for you to be moved here. And now that you're here, what difference does it make to you if we put these instruments on your body so the nurses can check on you without too much trouble?" The Rabbi told me that when he heard the doctor's words, he realised that he was seriously ill and the doctor was trying to encourage him with love and respect, so he would not be full of fear. The doctor's goodness had such an encouraging effect on him that he was completely cured in a very short time!

Perhaps this is the meaning of the Talmud's statement with which we began our article. It may well be that Heaven has decreed that a certain good doctor — and none other — using a certain good medicine, is indeed the agent chosen to effect the cure!

"Why Did You Save My Father's Life?"

HaRav Yitzchak Zilberstein,
Av Beit Din, Ramat Elchanan, Bnei Brak,
Rabbinical Committee of Laniado Hospital

Excerpts from an article in "Pathways in Medicine" 1 (Adar 5739 — March 1979).

Summary: Rabbi Zilberstein reminds us that even a person who appears to be on his deathbed may be saved by a miracle, and one should never give up hope or stop attempting to cure the patient.

An Orthodox cardiologist once told me about an incident that happened to him. He was called to the emergency ward to treat a patient whose breathing had stopped and who had been diagnosed as "clinically dead." The staff believed that he could be revived. After strenuous efforts, with the help of the Almighty, the doctor succeeded in bringing the patient back to life. Several days later, the sick man was even sitting up in bed! The doctor was visiting his patient, when by chance he met the sick man's son. Much to his surprise, and consternation, the son began to berate him. "My father is an incurably sick man," he said. "Why didn't you let him die in peace? Who asked you to bring him back to a life of suffering and pain? You have no conscience!"

The doctor told me that he had been expecting thanks from

the patient's relatives. Instead, he was subjected to a verbal attack! He asked me for advice on how to answer the sick man's son and refute the charges of causing unnecessary suffering and a lack of conscience.

I told him that the Rambam rules that any patient whose breathing has stopped is classed as a person who has lost consciousness, and, in such a case, the Torah obligates us to try to save his life. An example which illustrates the importance of this ruling can be found in the Tractate *Sofrim*, where there is a case of a person who had been declared dead, and then buried, only to rise from his grave and live for another twelve years, during which time he became the father of five children!

To appreciate the value the Torah places on saving a person's life, one should study the laws in the *Shulchan Aruch, Orach Chayim* 329. There a situation is described in which a man was partially buried beneath the earth in a landslide. His head was so badly injured that it was clear that at best he could only live a very short time. In such a case, Jewish Law states that, if necessary, the "whole of Israel should profane the Sabbath" to remove the earth and give the buried man a chance to live a little longer. According to Jewish Law, we are commanded to try to save a person's life, even if we think that he can only live a short time, and the short life remaining to him will be full of suffering.

He who saves a person's life, even for a short time, gives him an opportunity to repent.

A question connected with this case is raised by the *Bei'ur Halachah*: How can the "whole of Israel" be permitted to profane the Sabbath in order to save the buried person? We have been taught that the only reason one is allowed to profane the Sabbath is to save a life — that is, by profaning one Sabbath, one can ensure that many other Sabbaths will be observed. Since in this case the man is certain to die in a very short time, and almost certainly will not be able to observe one more Sabbath, how can "the whole of Israel" be permitted to profane the Sabbath in order to save him?

The *Bei'ur Halachah* answers that if the "whole of Israel" saves the buried man, even if he lives only a short time, he will still have time to repent over the fact that he has profaned many Sabbaths. This repentance will "put right" the many Sabbaths he has profaned, and he then can be regarded as if he were now in fact observing many Sabbaths — the Sabbaths which he profaned in the past, and has now succeeded in "putting right" through his repentance.

From this we many learn that a doctor who extends the life of a terminally ill patient even for a short time (even if the patient suffers), has performed a very good deed — he has given the sick man the opportunity to repent and "put right" his previous wrongdoings before he dies.

There is another point that should be considered. Our Rabbis explain that the conflict between righteousness and wickedness in the world can be thought of as a "balance" between good and evil. One additional righteous person could have the effect, unbeknownst to us, of "tipping the balance" in favour of righteousness. A man who is so seriously ill that he has only a short time to live can almost certainly be classed as a righteous person who is seeking to use the last moments of his life to put right his previous wrongdoings. If such a person is "saved" by a doctor, and given the opportunity to live a little longer, it is possible that this sick, but righteous, man will have power to tilt the balance in favour of righteousness in the world, and this could, perhaps, be described as having the effect of causing "many more Sabbaths to be observed."

The Talmud (*Yevamos* 121) cites several cases of people who, according to the laws of nature, should have died, but were saved to live long and fruitful lives. For example, the Talmud tells the story of a fisherman who disappeared under the water while laying his nets in the River Jordan, and was given up as dead. The following morning, he returned to his wife. He had entered a cave whose exit he had been unable to find until morning. The Talmud also relates an incident described by Rabbi Gamliel. During a sea voyage he noticed a sunken vessel, on which he knew that Rabbi Akiva had been a passenger. When Rabbi Gamliel reached the harbour, he was delighted and surprised to meet Rabbi Akiva, who sat with him and discussed the Torah. Rabbi Akiva explained that he had managed to hold onto a beam of the sunken vessel which had carried him to the dry land. In the same Tractate, Rabbi Akiva describes how he once saw a destroyed vessel, on which he knew Rabbi Meir had been a passenger. Later, Rabbi Meir described to Rabbi Akiva how he had been carried from wave to wave and washed up on the beach.

The Klausenberger Rav, *ztz"l*, has stated that Jewish Law, which obliges us to save a person whose head has been seriously injured, teaches us that even a seriously injured person can sometimes be completely cured, contrary to the laws of nature.

It is well known that doctors are sometimes amazed when they see a patient make a complete recovery, contrary to the laws of medicine and nature. Doctors know that not everything written in medical textbooks is sacred. In the course of their work, they experience many surprises and see many miracles!

In the case we referred to at the beginning of this article, the doctor should have answered the complaint of the sick man's son by reminding him that for each individual a miracle is possible. As the Talmud states in Tractate *Bava Kama* 2, a human being can sometimes recover from a blow that could kill an animal — not because a human being is stronger than an animal, but because a human being can be saved by Divine intervention, through Divine providence, and especially by the power of prayer which has been granted to him. The doctor should have told the son that our Torah commands us never to give up. A man's good deeds can protect him in his time of trouble, at the very moment when he appears to be on his deathbed.

Perhaps the doctor could have told the son the story of Binyamin HaTzaddik, quoted in *Bava Basra* 11. Binyamin HaTzaddik was in charge of distribution of charity to the poor. One day a lady came to him for help. He told her that to his sorrow the charity fund had no money left in it. The lady replied: "Rabbi, if you do not give me charity, a mother and her seven sons will die!" Binyamin HaTzaddik decided to support the lady and her sons with his own money. A little later, he fell seriously ill and was about to die. The Talmud relates that the Angels in Heaven said before the Heavenly Throne: "You have said that a person who saves one soul in Israel has saved a complete world. Binyamin HaTzaddik has saved a mother and her seven sons!" Immediately the decree of death that had been passed against him was rescinded, and he lived for another twenty-two years!

Operating on a Critically Ill Mother to Save a Fetus

HaRav Yitzchak Zilberstein,
Av Beit Din, Ramat Elchanan, Bnei Brak;
Rabbinical Committee of Laniado Hospital

Excerpts from an article in "Pathways in Medicine" 7 (Elul 5745 — September 1985).

Summary: Rabbi Zilberstein received a question from a hospital concerning a pregnant mother who was dangerously ill. The doctors asked whether they were allowed to perform a Caesarian operation on the mother in order to save the fetus, even if such an operation would seriously endanger the mother's life. Rabbi Zilberstein brings proofs from Jewish Law that the operation is not permissible, but if the mother's brain membranes were infected, a further question should be asked.

The following question was received from a hospital: "A forty-year-old woman has been admitted in the last trimester of her first pregnancy. She has been suffering for several weeks from a high temperature and headache. It is clear that she is suffering from encephalitis, a viral infection of the brain. Her condition has deteriorated, she has lost consciousness and it appears that there is little hope that she will survive. Her condition has been kept stablized with the help of liquid infusions, drugs and a breathing respirator. She is now in the ninth month of her pregnancy, and her condition is continuing to deteriorate. The question now is, how can the fetus be saved? While the viral infection has, in the main, attacked the mother, it is possible that it has also entered the womb, since there is evidence of infection in other parts of her body and in her blood. While one cannot rule out the possibility that the fetus has also been infected, examination indicates that the fetus is alive, and it appears to be perfectly well.

"Is it permissible to carry out a Caesarian section in order to save the fetus, as a spontaneous birth does not seem likely? It is impossible to predict how long the mother will live, and there is a danger that the opportunity to carry out the operation will be missed.

"The operation will not directly affect the mother, who appears to be approaching death. It is impossible, however, to ignore the fact that the operation will weaken her and could bring the day of her death nearer.

"Are we allowed to assume that if the mother were fully conscious she would agree to the operation?"

Our answer is based on several cardinal principles of Jewish Law.

In Tractate *Shabbos* 151, it is stated that one is forbidden to close the eyelids of a person who is very close to death, as the slightest pressure on that person's body could bring death nearer. Also the Rambam clearly states that one who deliberately kills a person who is on the brink of death is to be classified as a murderer.

The Rambam also states that one is not allowed to kill a Jewish person in order to save the life of another Jewish person.

Another basic principle of Jewish Law is "a human being is not the owner, or the master, of his own body." Thus a Jewish man cannot be put to death solely because he confesses to a capital crime, but only on the testimony of two witnesses. "The soul of a man is not his own possession, but a possession of his Creator. His confession has no relevance: it concerns a body which does not belong to him" (Radbaz).

Based on the above, it appears that it is forbidden to perform an operation on the mother who is approaching death, in order to save the fetus; it is forbidden to kill, or even bring nearer to death, a person on the verge of death. This prohibition applies even if the intention is to save another life. In this case, the prohibition appears to be even stronger. There is no certainty that the fetus will survive the operation, especially since there is a risk that the fetus itself has become infected with the mother's illness.

In the *Shulchan Aruch, Orach Chayim* 330, we find the following law: "In the case of a pregnant mother who has died during childbirth, one is obligated to carry a knife through the public domain on the Sabbath in order to operate on her and save the fetus." But the Rema adds: "We must not even carry the knife on a weekday, because there is no one expert enough to decide the exact moment when the mother has already died and the child is still alive."

A case has been cited where a pregnant mother was told by her doctors that if her pregnancy were allowed to continue, she would almost certainly die, and he advised her to have an abortion at once. The mother refused to allow the abortion to be performed. She said that she would rather die than allow her child to be killed. From this it appears that a mother has the right to virtually "kill herself" in order to save the life of her fetus.

This case is slightly different from the case we are considering. In this case, the mother did not actively consent to an operation, which could kill her, in order to save the child in her womb. All she asked was that the doctors do nothing but allow the pregnancy to take its usual course. In the case we are considering, the doctors ask if they can operate on the mother in order to save the fetus.

Another relevant point must be considered. An expert gynaecologist stated that, in this case, after the fortieth week of pregnancy the mother's placenta would rapidly age and deteriorate very quickly, and if birth did not take place, complications would certainly ensue which would cause the mother's death.

From this, it might appear that an operation would be permissible and obligatory, in spite of all the risks involved, to save the mother's life and the life of the fetus. This, however, is on the condition that the pregnancy has already reached the forty-second week, when the placenta begins to deteriorate, and the operation could be permitted as a means of saving life.

Similarly, should the mother begin to feel contractions which could endanger her life, then a Caesarian operation could be carried out in spite of the risks involved, as such an operation would not be causing death, but an attempt to save life.

There is a final point to be considered which may furnish some slight grounds for performing the operation. If the virus has taken such a strong hold on the mother that her brain membranes have been infected with meningitis, then she could be classed as a person "certain to die." This would render her a *treifah* in Jewish Law. The Rambam states (*Hilchos Roze'ach U'Shemiras Nefesh* 2:8) that a person who kills a *treifah* is not liable to suffer the death sentence. (The Meiri adds that the person is liable to a death sentence "in the eyes of Heaven.")

A relevant case is to be found in Tractate *Nedarim* 22. There we are told how Ulla was travelling to the Land of Israel accompanied by two men. One of the men suddenly stabbed the other, and while the injured man was in the throes of his last dying struggles, the murderer turned to Ulla and said: "See what a wonderful thing I have done!" The Talmud states that Ulla said to the murderer: "You have done a good job. Now go and finish the work." This difficult passage is usually explained in the following manner. As the dying man was a *treifah,* and in his last death struggles, Ulla had considered it permissible to say these words in order to save his own life. From this we might conclude that if the mother's brain membranes have been infected with meningitis, in which case she would be classed as a *treifah* — one who is certain to die — perhaps the operation to save the life of the fetus would be permitted.

One can also take into account the fact that it is not certain that the operation will cause her death. In addition, perhaps the mother would have agreed to the operation had she been conscious.

In the light of all the matters considered above, I sent the following answer to the doctors who put the question to me:

1. No permission can be given to perform the operation on the mother in order to save the fetus if the operation could bring the death of the mother nearer. Even if the mother agreed to the operation, her agreement would not be relevant.

2. In the case of a pregnancy which endangers the life of the mother, an abortion can be performed in order to save her life. On the other hand, if the mother refuses to agree to the abortion, her wishes must be respected, and it should not be carried out.

3. In the case we are considering, if the placenta is rapidly aging and thus endangering the life of the mother, permission could be granted to carry out the operation, which would have the aim of saving the mother's life, and secondly the life of the fetus.

4. If the infection has already reached the membranes of the mother's brain, and the mother is therefore "certain to die," there are some Rabbis who might consider the possibility of allowing the operation to take place, but this would require further consideration before permission could be given.

Violating the Sabbath for One Who Has Deliberately Endangered His Life

HaRav Gabriel Zinner,
Dayan, Beth She'arim Community, New York

Excerpts from an article in "Pathways in Medicine" 8 (Kislev 5747 — January 1987).

Summary: Rabbi Zinner asks if it is permissible to profane the Sabbath to save the life of a Jewish person who has deliberately harmed himself, by, for example, trying to commit suicide. He quotes various sources which could support the argument that the Sabbath should not be violated in order to cure such a person. However, he concludes that the accepted view of the Torah is that one must profane the Sabbath in order to save the life of such a person.

Question:

Is it permissible to violate the Sabbath in order to save the life of someone who has deliberately and wrongfully placed his life in danger?

Answer:

In Tractate *Yoma* 85 there is a ruling that one should profane the Sabbath in order to save the life of another person, even if that person is only likely to live for a very short time. One may well ask why it is permitted to violate the Sabbath to heal a person who is only likely to live for a very short time. The reason given for this permission is that one should "profane one Sabbath so that many Sabbaths will be kept." If so, how can we violate the Sabbath to save the life of a person who will only live for an hour or two? How will such a person be able to "keep many Sabbaths"? The Meiri explains that the reason for this ruling is that it may well be that in the short time left to him, the person will repent and confess his wrongdoings.

Our original question still remains. If the purpose of violating the Sabbath to save a person is to give that person a chance to carry out the commandments of the Torah and lead a spiritual life, even for a short time, how can it be permissible to profane the Sabbath to save the life of a disbeliever who has deliberately and wrongfully put his own life in danger? The reason given for violating the Sabbath in order to save a life is that the commandments of the Torah are given to us in order "to live by them," and not to "die by them." But, "to live by them" is, as we have seen, explained by the Rabbis as "living a spiritual life" in order to gain one's reward in the World to Come. If so, how can the Sabbath be violated in order to save the life of a disbeliever?

Once when I was discussing this problem with the Grand Rabbi of Sanz, *ztz"l,* he pointed out that the Torah does suggest that mercy is not shown to a person who has put himself in danger, since a person who has no understanding is not worthy of mercy. The Grand Rabbi of Sanz, *ztz"l,* explained to me that this only refers to a person who begs for mercy through prayer, but certainly one should use medical means to heal such a person, as we are forbidden to merely watch without acting when our brother is suffering. Furthermore, a Jew is commanded to restore to another Jew a possession which he has lost. We must, therefore, strive to restore another Jew to life, even by profaning the Sabbath.

However, it appears to me that it may be possible to learn from an event described in Tractate *Yoma* 85 that one should not violate the Sabbath in order to save a person who has wrongfully placed himself in danger. The Talmud there tells the story of Hillel HaZaken who climbed on the roof of the house of study and listened through a window to the words of Torah expounded by Shemaya and Avtalyon. He had climbed onto the roof just before a Sabbath in the winter. During the night, there was a heavy snowfall, which completey covered Hillel. In the morning, Shemaya and Avtalyon noticed the figure of a man outlined against the skylight. The Talmud relates that the two Rabbis carried Hillel down from the roof, broke the ice off him, washed him, rubbed him down and placed him in front of the fire. All this was done on the Sabbath, and the Rabbis said: "*This* person is worthy to have the Sabbath profaned for him."

This statement requires explanation. Could it be that only Hillel was worthy to have the Sabbath profaned for him? Is not every Jew worthy to be treated in this way? Hillel had acted wrongly. He should have come down from the roof as soon as the snow began to fall. He himself brought about the circumstance which had led to the profanation of the Sabbath. The Talmud explains that Hillel's love of Torah was so strong that he did not even feel the snow and ice. He did not act wrongly. He had entered into a dangerous situation unintentionally. Perhaps we may learn from this that if a person deliberately and knowingly endangers his life, he is not worthy, and the Sabbath should not be profaned in order to cure him.

In fact, this is not the view accepted by the Torah. A famous Rabbi cites the case of a young girl who drank poison, and he reports that the Chida ruled that it was necessary to profane the Sabbath to save her life.

Another great Rabbi rules that it is quite clear that a person who has attempted to commit suicide must be saved, even if it is necessary to profane the Sabbath, because a person's "life does not belong to him, but is the possession of his Creator." Similarly, the Rabbis also state that one is forbidden to strike a blow at another person, even if that person has asked him to do it. No one has the authority to ask another person to harm his body, which is not his possession, but belongs to Hashem. Similarly, the Rambam states that the reason a person cannot be put to death or legally punished on the basis of his own testimony is that a person's life is not his own possession, but the possession of his Creator. One is therefore obligated to strive to heal a person who attempts suicide, because he cannot be considered to be a person who has deliberately and carelessly lost something that belongs to him. Rather he is comparable to someone who has lost something that belongs to someone else, and we are, therefore, obliged to strive to restore the lost object to its real owner.

A person who deliberately puts himself into danger should be given treatment and healed, even if the Sabbath has to be profaned. We are instructed to compel a sick person to eat on the Day of Atonement if his doctor advises it, even though he may not wish to do so. A person does not own his own body. His body is a possession of the Creator, and it is our duty to strive to heal and protect Hashem's possessions.

In conclusion, one must profane the Sabbath to heal a person who has deliberately caused his illness and is in danger of dying.

Abortion in the First Forty Days

HaRav Aharon Wieder,
Rabbinical Court of Sanz, Brooklyn, New York

Excerpts from an article in "Pathways in Medicine" 2(Elul 5739 — September 1979).

Summary: Rabbi Wieder concludes that a fetus must be considered a living entity even in the first forty days of pregnancy. Therefore, abortion must be considered forbidden according to Biblical Law, even in the first forty days of pregnancy.

In the first volume of the journal *Pathways in Medicine*, the great Rabbi and Gaon, Rabbi Yitzchak Zilberstein, discussed the prohibition of abortion in Jewish Law, and mentioned that there is a difference between the first forty days of pregnancy and the remaining period of the pregnancy, since there are some Rabbis who hold that an abortion during the first forty days is only forbidden by rabbinical decree, not by a Biblical prohibition. Their reason is that they don't consider the fetus (during the first forty days of pregnancy) to be a living entity, but is comparable to water. After forty days, the fetus has developed, and an abortion would then be forbidden by Biblical Law. I would like to comment on this subject.

In Tractate *Yevamos* 69, a case is discussed where the daughter of a Kohen marries a Yisroel. Her husband dies before she has any children. The Talmud states that she may eat *terumah* immediately, that very evening. Rav Chisdah questions this opinion, stating that she may eat the *terumah* at any time up to forty days after the death of her husband. The reason he gives is that if she were pregnant when her husband died (which would make her eating *terumah* forbidden), then during the first forty days of pregnancy she should not be considered as being truly pregnant, since until forty days after conception the fetus is only regarded as if it were water.

From this discussion it might appear that an abortion is not forbidden by Biblical Law during the first forty days of pregnancy. But this may not be the correct conclusion. All that we can conclude from the discussion in Tractate *Yevamos* is that until forty days have passed since conception, the daughter of a Kohen married to a Yisroel who died is permitted to eat *terumah*. We cannot conclude from this that before forty days have passed, the fetus is comparable to water in every respect.

Some support can be found for the proposition that the fetus must be regarded as an actual fetus from the moment of conception from Tractate *Sotah* 2. Rabbi Yehuda is quoted as saying that forty days before the formation of the fetus, a voice calls out from Heaven saying: "The daughter of this person shall marry this person." The Maharshah explains the words of Rabbi Yehuda in the following way: "Forty days before the formation of the embryo" refers to to the moment of conception. According to this view, at the very beginning of the pregnancy, even before forty days have passed, the male is already a fetus. It is not to be considered as merely water, since the name of its future spouse was already called out by a Heavenly voice.

The Rabbinical commentators also discuss a case cited in the *Shulchan Aruch* of a man who gives a gift to a fetus. The gift is binding if the fetus is the donor's own child. The reasoning behind this decision is that a person is attached to his own child, and therefore the gift has been donated with a strong intention. Here the Rabbis make no distinction between the first forty days of pregnancy and the rest of the pregnancy. The father's gift is binding even if it is given at the very beginning of the pregnancy. The Rabbis do not say that the gift is only binding if forty days of the pregnancy have passed, as the fetus is merely water before that time.

I have found a report of an actual case which came before the Rabbinical Court of the town of Lonil. A person had given a gift to his child while it was still in the womb — during the first forty days of the pregnancy. It is recorded that the Rabbinical Court was divided in its opinion. Some members of the court held that the gift was not valid, as it was given during the first forty days of pregnancy, when the fetus was still to be considered as if it were merely water. Other members of the Court held that the gift was binding on the donor, since a man has a special feeling towards his own child even when it is in the womb, and the fetus must be considered to be such from the very beginning of the pregnancy. The Rabbinical Court decided, according to the majority opinion, that the gift was binding and the fetus must be considered a living fetus during the first forty days of the pregnancy.

However, one still hesitates to draw the conclusion from this case that an abortion before forty days after conception is forbidden according to Biblical Law, since we are considering the "feelings" of the donor towards his own future offspring. Perhaps the actual state of the fetus in this connection is not completely relevant.

The Talmud suggests another distinction:

Within the first forty days, a fetus may be considered such from the point of view of the father. However, from the point of view of the mother, it may be considered merely water. At this stage it is comparable to a limb of the mother which has not developed enough to be called a separate being. This is why, referring to the case we quoted in Tractate *Yevamos*, the mother is allowed to eat the priestly food in the first forty days of her pregnancy. During this time, from her point of view, the fetus may be compared to water. It is not yet a separate being.

There are many opinions in the Talmud which state that the Sabbath and the Day of Atonement should be profaned to save the life of a fetus, even during the first forty days of pregnancy. If the fetus is regarded merely as water, it surely would not be permissible to profane the Sabbath and the Day of Atonement to save its life.

Again, in Tractate *Sanhedrin* there is a discussion on the question of the exact point in time when the soul of a person enters the body. One opinion holds that the soul enters the body at the moment when the Angel "visits the first drop of life," which would mean that life exists in the fetus from the first moment of pregnancy. Another opinion is that the soul enters the body at the "moment of the creation of the fetus." This could mean when the fetus already had some sinew and bone, only after forty days have elapsed. The Talmud accepts the first point of view: the soul enters the embryo at the first moment of pregnancy; it becomes a complete, living embryo from that very first moment.

In conclusion: from a consideration of all the material, one must conclude that an abortion during the first forty days of pregnancy must be considered to be forbidden according to Biblical Law, and that in cases of abortion no distinction should be made between before and after forty days of pregnancy.

Treating a Patient on Yom Kippur

HaRav Shmuel Baruch Werner,
Chief Dayan, Rabbinical Court of Tel Aviv

Excerpts from an article in "Pathways in Medicine" 1 (Adar 5739 — March 1979).

Summary: Rabbi Werner considers several problems that arise in connection with a sick person who has to eat on Yom Kippur for health reasons.

A sick person is permitted to eat on Yom Kippur if his life would be endangered by fasting

Jewish Law clearly states that a dangerously ill person should be given food on Yom Kippur if a doctor so prescribes, or if the sick person himself feels that he would be endangering his life if he fasted. Moreover, even if a doctor states that the person would not die if he fasted, but his illness would worsen, he may not fast. The Talmud derives this law from *VaYikra* 18:5, which states: "Ye shall therefore keep My statutes, and My ordinances, which if a man do, he shall live by them." On this verse the Talmud comments: "You shall live by them and not die by them."

The Jerusalem Talmud (*Yoma,* chap. 8) states that a person who acts quickly when a patient's life is in danger is worthy of praise. It adds that a person who delays the treatment of a dangerously ill patient in order to ask a Rabbi as to whether or not such a person is permitted to eat on Yom Kippur or whether one may violate the Sabbath on his behalf, is guilty of shedding the other person's blood, while the Rabbi to whom the questions were put deserves rebuke. The commentators explain that the Rabbi deserves rebuke because he should have taught his congregation and made it perfectly clear to them that both the Sabbath and Yom Kippur *must* be profaned when there is a danger to life.

What if the doctors disagree with each other over the seriousness of the patient's illness?

If one doctor says that a patient should eat on Yom Kippur, and another doctor says that he should not eat, we must follow the advice of the doctor who says he should eat, since when life is in danger we must always act leniently. The Rabbis tell us that if two doctors say that the patient should not eat, and one says that he should eat, we follow the advice of the doctors who say he should not eat. However, if the doctor who says he should eat is a greater expert than the other two doctors, we follow the advice of the greater expert and allow the patient to eat. There is a discussion among the Rabbis about how to act in a situation where there is a difference of opinion among the doctors, but, in general, greater weight is given to the opinion of the doctor who is recognised to have the greater expertise.

What if the doctors order the patient to eat on Yom Kippur but he refuses to do so?

The Ramban states that if a sick person wishes to fast on

Yom Kippur and it will put his life in danger, he is by no means acting in a pious fashion and could, in fact, deserve serious punishment. The Radvaz says that such a person is classed as a "stupid religious fanatic." He is comparable to one who has shed blood, and he will surely be severely punished by Hashem.

It should be added that some Rabbis maintain that a doctor is only permitted to heal external injuries. According to this opinion, a doctor should not treat internal illnesses; these should be left entirely to Hashem to heal. According to this view, it would be permissible for a patient to refuse to accept the doctor's instruction to eat on Yom Kippur if his illness were internal and not external.

Not all Rabbis, however, agree that this opinion should be followed in practice. Moreover, there is a clear opinion nowadays that the treatment of internal illness also falls within the province of the doctor, since the use of X-rays and other modern methods of diagnosis allows the doctor to treat an internal illness in the same way as he would treat external disorders.

Thus we can see that there is agreement among the Rabbis that a patient is forbidden to ignore the instructions of the doctor. In this connection I wish to quote the words of the great Rabbi Shmuel Bornstein, of blessed memory, who once wrote to his sick son-in-law as follows: "May Hashem soon restore you to your former health. Now Yom Kippur is fast approaching. I warn you not to be over-righteous about fasting. Whatever the doctors tell you to do, you must do. If they tell you that you should eat, but only small quantities, then eat an amount equivalent to half the size of an egg within a period of eight minutes. However, if they tell you that this would not be enough for you, then Heaven forbid that you should be hard upon yourself! For He who ordered you to fast upon Yom Kippur also ordered you to obey the doctors when they tell you *not* to fast. In no circumstances should you feel that the permission to eat on Yom Kippur is only for a very seriously ill person. Heaven forbid! When it comes to risks to health, we are lenient even when there is the slightest doubt. You surely remember what I have told you so many times. One of the basic principles of Judaism is that a man should nullify his own will, so that he acts only according to the laws of the Torah and to the rulings of the Rabbis, even if they tell him that right is left! Therefore, do not be upset if you do not fast on Yom Kippur, because if you listen to the words of the Rabbis who tell you to obey the doctors when they tell you not to fast, you will be given a greater reward than if you actually fasted. Therefore, eat with a happy heart. Eat your bread and drink your wine cheerfully, because Hashem recognises that your actions are good deeds."

It is quite clear that our Rabbis rule that it is forbidden to be strict with oneself and fast when the doctors have ordered one not to fast. The Rabbis even go further and state that a person who obstinately refuses to eat when the doctors have instructed him to do so should be forced to eat against his will. The Rabbis add, however, that if the patient fears that eating, or taking a certain medicine, will harm him, then he should not be forced to eat or take the medicine. For example, if a patient says that he does not wish to suffer any more and prefers to die, we do not listen to him, but do all we can to save his life, even against his will: the Torah commands us that it is forbidden to stand idly by while our neighbour is in danger of losing his life. In this case, the opinion of the sick man is not relevant. He has no right to destroy himself. However, if a person who suffers from severe pain wishes to undergo an operation to relieve the pain, he is permitted to do so, even though the operation may prove fatal, since there is a good chance that the operation will succeed and the pain be alleviated. Nevertheless, a person is duty-bound not to take undue risks, and if the pain he is suffering from does not constitute a risk to his life, it would be better if he did not undergo a risky operation, but continued to suffer pain in the hope that his condition would heal on its own. Actually, we rule that a person should not undergo an operation which could endanger his life without consulting three doctors. Of course, in emergency cases, where there is no time to seek such opinions, the operation should be performed as soon as possible.

From this discussion, the following question arises. How can surgeons operate on a person against his will? Surely a man is master of his own body. He alone should decide what is to be done with his body and whether he should live or die. Who should be more in charge of a man's body than the man himself?

The answer is clear. The Torah tells us that a man is *not* in charge of his own body and *not* the master of his own soul. His soul is the property of the Creator of all souls. It is part of the Divine Spirit, and a man is not its owner. A man is, therefore, forbidden to commit suicide. The Rabbis state that a person who deliberately chokes himself is comparable to a murderer.

Just as it is forbidden to destroy oneself, it is forbidden to refuse treatment that could save oneself from death. If a sick person refuses treatment that could save him, he should be given the treatment against his will, and even operated on against his will, in order to save a life. Thus, in the original case under discussion — if a sick person refuses to eat on Yom Kippur, even though the doctors have instructed him to do so — we are permitted to feed him forcibly without his consent.

A sick person who eats on Yom Kippur need not feel that he has committed a sin. On the contrary, he has carried out a commandment of the Torah that tells us we must protect our lives. There are those who remind us of the statement in the Talmud that if we do not eat in the Sukkah during Sukkot because it is raining, we should feel like a servant who brought his master a glass of water, and the master threw it back in the servant's face instead of drinking it. It has been suggested that a sick person who eats on Yom Kippur should feel like that servant. But this comparison only applies to the Sukkah, not to other situations where a person *apparently* does not fulfil a commandment. And even in the case of the Sukkah, this applies only when it rains — not if a person cannot eat in the Sukkah for some other reason, such as sickness.

Is a person who eats on Yom Kippur obligated to say a blessing and mention "Yom Kippur" in the Grace after Meals?

A sick person who eats on Yom Kippur is obligated to say the blessings both before and after eating. The situation is not comparable to a person who eats forbidden food, and, according to some opinions, should not say blessings. The sick person who eats on Yom Kippur is permitted to eat the food.

Our Rabbis are divided in their opinions as to whether or not the day, "Yom Kippur," should be mentioned in the Grace after Meals recited by a sick person. All agree that if a sick person does mention "Yom Kippur" in the section *Ya'aleh VeYavo* in the Grace after Meals, it is not considered to be an interruption in the prayer.

Should a sick person who has to eat on Yom Kippur recite Kiddush before eating?

Our Rabbis also discuss the problem of whether or not a person who is permitted to eat on Yom Kippur should recite Kiddush before he eats. The Magen Avraham holds that it is preferable not to recite Kiddush on Yom Kippur; one may be reciting an unnecessary blessing, which is not permissible. Rabbi Akiva Eger writes that the Magen Avraham may be referring to a situation when Yom Kippur falls on a weekday, in which case the obligation to recite Kiddush is Rabbinical, not Biblical. But the situation may be different if Yom Kippur falls on the Sabbath, when there is a Biblical obligation to recite Kiddush. In this connection, it is recorded that the great Rabbi Nahum Ze'ev Borenstein, of blessed memory, asked his young son (who was not obligated to fast) if he had recited Kiddush before he ate on Yom Kippur morning. His son, who was later to become a great Rabbi himself, answered that he had recited the blessing over wine, which may be regarded as equivalent to Kiddush. From this we may conclude that the son was referring to a case where Yom Kippur fell on a weekday. If the incident had occurred when Yom Kippur coincided with the Sabbath, the son would have been obligated to recite the whole of the Friday night Kiddush in the morning, since he had clearly not recited it the previous evening, as a young boy normally does not eat on the evening of Yom Kippur, but waits until morning to break his fast.

From this discussion it appears clear to me that if Yom Kippur falls on a weekday, there is no obligation to recite a full Kiddush. However, if Yom Kippur falls on the Sabbath, and Kiddush was not said in the evening because the fast had not been broken yet, it appears that the full Friday-night Kiddush should be recited on Yom Kippur morning when a person eats.

Is a sick person who has eaten on Yom Kippur permitted to eat during the rest of the day, even if he is no longer dangerously ill?

The question has been asked: can a sick person who has eaten once on Yom Kippur continue to eat during the rest of the day, even if he is no longer in serious danger? The question is, is the commandment "to afflict oneself" on Yom Kippur binding through the day, or if, after one has already broken the fast, the commandment "to afflict oneself" may no longer be applicable on that Yom Kippur? The answer to this question is given in one of the Responsa of the Chasam Sofer. He was asked if a person who had eaten on Yom Kippur because of illness could be called to the reading of the Torah on the afternoon of Yom Kippur, since only people who are fasting can be called to the Torah on a fast day. He replied that such a person can be called to the reading of the Torah "since he is not obligated to fast." However, the Chasam Sofer emphasises that in such a case, a sick person is only permitted to eat an amount sufficient to revive him and remove the danger to his life. He clearly states that if a drink would be sufficient to put him out of danger, he should not eat. If eating once would put him out of danger, he should not eat twice. If he follows these rulings, he is to be regarded as if he had actually fasted, and he may be called to the reading of the Torah.

The author of *Aruch LeNair* makes the same point. He quotes Rashi and the Tosephos in Tractate *Yoma*, who write that the punishment given to a person who eats on Yom Kippur (*kores*) still applies *after* a person has eaten once on that day for reasons of health. If a person has eaten on Yom Kippur morning because of his health, and eats again on Yom Kippur afternoon even though he is out of danger, he is liable for the punishment for eating on Yom Kippur. One must conclude that on Yom Kippur a sick person should only eat enough food to remove the danger to his life, and no more. It is a most difficult task to measure this quantity exactly, and I am very surprised that our great Rabbis have not emphasised this point more, in view of the gravity of the sin of eating unnecessarily on Yom Kippur.

Kiddush recited by a sick person on a Yom Kippur that falls on the Sabbath should not be recited over wine

From the preceding discussion, we may derive an additional point. We have learned that it appears that a person who has to eat on a Yom Kippur that falls on a Sabbath should recite Kiddush before eating. There is, however, no necessity to drink wine after reciting the Kiddush, as one would not normally require wine to remove a danger to his life. He should recite the Kiddush over bread, and then eat the minimum amount that is absolutely necessary to remove the danger.

Treatment of Non-Jewish Patients

HaRav Moshe Sternbuch,
Rosh Yeshiva, Yeshivat Rosh Ha'ayin

Extracts from an article in "Pathways in Medicine" 6 (Elul 5744 — September 1984).

Summary: Rabbi Sternbuch considers whether or not a Jewish doctor is permitted to approve the "mercy killing" of a *non-Jewish,* critically ill patient. ("Mercy-killing" of a *Jewish* patient is in every case classified as murder.) He then goes on to discuss the problems faced by the Jewish doctor in his treatment of non-Jewish patients, both in hospital and privately, and whether or not he is permitted to violate the Sabbath in order to treat a non-Jewish patient.

In Johannesburg, I was once asked a question by a religious Jewish doctor who held the position of Director of a non-Jewish hospital. One of the patients in the hospital was a critically ill non-Jew who had only a short time to live and was in intense pain. Both he and his close relatives had begged the doctors treating him to have mercy on him by giving him drugs which would cause his speedy death. The doctors agreed to the suggestion, but could not carry it out until they received an authority to do so signed by the Director of the hospital. The Director, a religious Jew, was very hesitant to sign this authority. He knew that the patient was a non-Jew and that "mercy-killing" was permissible according to non-Jewish law in South Africa, but perhaps it was not permissible according to the Torah. According to the Torah, a non-Jew is forbidden to kill another non-Jew, even if the victim at the time of his death is already fatally ill, and, according to the Torah, a non-Jew who kills another non-Jew is liable to the death penalty. The doctor reasoned, if a non-Jew is not permitted to kill another non-Jew according to the Torah, then a Jew certainly would not be permitted to do so. As the Talmud in Tractate *Chullin* asks: "How can an action which is forbidden for a non-Jew be permissible for a Jew?" In addition, the doctor knew that a Jew is forbidden to cause a non-Jew to sin unwittingly. The Torah forbids him "to place a stumbling block before a blind man." For all these reasons, he hesitated before signing the authority, but he was concerned that if he continued to refuse to sign it, his career prospects would be harmed. Nevertheless, he asked me for a ruling according to the Torah.

In this connection, I recalled a story told of Rabbi Chayim of Brisk. One Rosh HaShanah he was called by the police to visit a Jew in a non-Jewish prison who had been condemned to death on a charge of murder. The authorities wished to give the condemned man the opportunity to confess his sins to the Rabbi of the town before he died, and for this reason they asked the Rabbi of Brisk to visit him without delay. The Rabbi realised that if he hurried to the prison, as the authorities wished, he would in fact be hastening the prisoner's death. He, therefore, made up every excuse he could in order to delay his visit. He did manage to delay the execution, and, by a miracle, the execution did not take place; it was suddenly postponed by the authorities. From this story, one might reason that the doctor who had asked me for the ruling should adopt similar tactics and delay his signing of the authority on some pretext in order to postpone the killing of the patient!

In fact, according to the Torah, the prohibition against killing a non-Jew is very strict. The Torah states that he who sheds the blood of another man will have his own blood shed by another, and this statement applies to a Jew who kills a non-Jew as well.

However, according to Jewish Law, there are some considerations which could allow the doctor to sign the authority requested from him. The Rabbis in our generation have considered the question of whether in our day non-Jews should be considered to be in the same category as the "idol-worshippers" of Biblical days. They generally come to the conclusion that the non-Jew in our day could be considered an idol-worshipper. Now, according to the Torah, an idol-worshipper is deserving of death. One could suggest that, in this case, since the Jewish doctor is not actually administering the drugs himself (but only giving permission to his non-Jewish associates to accede to the patient's own request that they kill him) and since the patient could perhaps be classed as an "idol-worshipper" who is deserving of death, a Rabbi may give the Jewish doctor permission to sign the authority. One could also say that the strict prohibition against killing a non-Jew refers to an actual killing in a cruel manner, and may well not apply to a case of "mercy-killing" done out of love for the patient, where the Jewish doctor himself would not carry out any physical action in a cruel manner.

In fact, I gave the Jewish doctor permission to sign the authority. I came to this conclusion especially when I took into consideration the fact that the patient had been diagnosed as fatally ill, with only a very short time to live in any case, as some Rabbis are of the opinion that killing a non-Jew who is on the point of dying need not always be classified as murder.

I also bore in mind the fact that in this hospital there were no Jewish patients — only non-Jews — and non-Jewish law actually permitted "mercy-killing" of this nature. However, I wish to make it clear that if this had taken place in a hospital that treated both Jewish and non-Jewish patients, in no circumstances could permission be granted to the Jewish doctor to sign the authority. A Jewish doctor working in such a "mixed" hospital may not be given permission to assist in the "mercy-killing" of a non-Jewish patient, because there is grave risk that other people, at a later date, will seek to prove from his action that "mercy-killing" can also be performed in the case of Jewish patients. "Mercy-killing" of a Jewish patient by a Jewish doctor is, without doubt, classified as murder. Similarly, if there happens to be a non-Jewish patient in a Jewish hospital, it is forbidden to accede to his request for a "mercy-killing." It should be made clear to all in a Jewish hospital that such an act is out of the question.

Some Rabbis have given permission to doctors to violate the Sabbath to save the life of a non-Jewish patient. It seems to me that such permission can only be made use of in hospitals where there are Jewish and non-Jewish patients; in such a hospital, a Jewish doctor who refuses to violate the Sabbath in order to help a non-Jewish patient, but is willing to do so in order to help a Jewish patient, would be bound to cause hatred towards the Jews, which would be dangerous to Jews. If the hospital in which the Jewish doctor is working has *only* non-Jewish patients, it would be completely forbidden for the Jewish doctor to violate the Sabbath in order to help the non-Jewish patients. How could any Rabbi give a Jewish doctor permission to work in a non-Jewish hospital where there are no Jewish patients and violate the Sabbath there? In such a case, the Jewish doctor would have to be classed as a Jew who violates the Sabbath *intentionally*. As the Rambam writes in *Hilchos Yesodei HaTorah*: "If he could escape from the dictates of a cruel King who orders him to violate the Sabbath, and does *not* escape intentionally, he may be compared to a dog wallowing in his own filth and is classed as an idol-worshipper, who loses his right to be in Heaven and descends to the lowest depths of Hell." If the doctor works in a hospital where there are both Jewish and non-Jewish patients, he must violate the Sabbath to treat the Jewish patients, and he is given special permission to violate the Sabbath for non-Jews, for if he does not do so he will arouse the hatred of the non-Jews towards the Jews.

Permission for a Jewish doctor to violate the Sabbath to treat a non-Jew is only to be given in exceptional cases, out of fear that a refusal to do so will cause dangerous anti-semitism. The permission may be compared to a ruling which the great Rabbi Yisroel Salanter gave in 1860. A terrible epidemic of cholera struck Vilna, and many Jews were infected. Rabbi Yisroel Salanter ruled that every Jew in Vilna, whether he was sick or not, should eat on the Day of Atonement. The situation was so serious that the ruling was based solely on the need to save Jewish lives: if some Jews who were not sick fasted on Yom Kippur, many who were sick would also fast, and, under the medical conditions in those days, they would certainly die. Rabbi Yisroel Salanter knew that in order to save the lives of the many Jews who would literally kill themselves by fasting, he had to issue a general permission for *all* the Jews in Vilna to eat on the Day of Atonement. Similarly, a Jewish doctor is only permitted to violate the Sabbath to help a non-Jewish patient if the consequences of his not doing so would be catastrophic to other Jews, as a result of the hatred that would be aroused among non-Jews. This does not give permission to a Jewish doctor to violate the Sabbath to save the life of a non-Jew in a place where there are no other Jews, or in a hospital where there are only non-Jews. In such a case, he has no authority to transgress the rulings of the Torah. He is under no compulsion to treat non-Jewish patients there on the Sabbath.

It is well known that Jewish doctors who have just qualified are required to work for a period of time in a hospital, and they sometimes have to work during this period in a non-Jewish hospital where there are no Jewish patients. In these circumstances, recently qualified Jewish doctors perform many tasks that transgress the Sabbath, such as drawing blood for tests. In fact, such tasks are usually put into the hands of newly-qualified doctors. In my opinion, for this reason, Jewish doctors are not permitted in any way to complete their training period in non-Jewish hospitals. They should certainly try to arrange to complete their training in religious hospitals in Israel, where there is no risk of wrongfully violating the Sabbath.

In fact, the permission given to a Jewish doctor to violate the Sabbath on behalf of a non-Jewish patient cannot be given easily, and in such cases it is always preferable, if possible, to ask a non-Jew to carry out the prohibited actions. Even in the case of private doctors, I have often advised them to come to an arrangement with a non-Jewish doctor, who should attend their patients on the Sabbath while the Jewish doctor in return looks after the patients of the non-Jewish doctor on Sunday. I have found that this arrangement often works very well, and certainly cannot cause any hatred of the non-Jew towards the Jew.

Those doctors who claim that they have full permission to violate the Sabbath in order to heal non-Jews, and work regularly in this fashion Sabbath after Sabbath, in my opinion are acting very wrongly, and have no permission to do this. If a doctor is faced with such a situation, he should rather travel to Israel and work there among Jewish people in a religious hospital which is ruled by the Laws of the Torah.

I would like to add that even if the doctor is treating a Jew, for whom he is permitted to violate the Sabbath, and he knows that he will have to visit him on the Sabbath, he should make arrangements to stay over in the hospital for the Sabbath, or near the hospital, so that he thus avoids violating the Sabbath. In this way he will receive the reward both for healing a sick patient and also for sanctifying the holy Sabbath.

Jewish Medical Care in Tiberias 1892 — 1896

Yisroel Freidin

Summary: Mr Freidin presents an account of the fascinating, poignant story of the struggles and efforts of the small Jewish community of Tiberias to establish a Jewish hospital in their town approximately a hundred years ago.

In Tractate *Pesachim* 8, it is stated: "Rabbi Dostoei, the son of Rabbi Yannai, said: Why were the hot springs of Tiberias not located in Jerusalem? So that the pilgrims to Jerusalem should not say: 'Even if we had only come to Jerusalem in order to bathe in the hot springs, it would have been sufficient,' and thus the holy motivation of their pilgrimage to Jerusalem would have been corrupted."

Thus the words of the great Rabbi Dostoei, a pupil of Rabbi Meir Baal HaNess who, is buried near the hot springs of Tiberias, give us some of idea of the veneration that was felt for the hot springs of Tiberias in ancient times. The great medical benefits to be obtained from bathing in the hot springs of Tiberias were thus well known already in ancient times. However, a study of their history during the last two hundred years reveals that their beneficial powers were not always utilised to full effect.

The first modern medical clinic was established in Tiberias in the year 1871. A newspaper of that time reports that a religious charity group interested in the care of the sick had been given the use of four rooms by the leaders of the religious

Ashkenazi community in Tiberias. The names of the three leaders mentioned were Rabbi Avraham Josef Alter HaLevy, the head of the Talmudical Acadamy of Vahlin, Rabbi Mordechai Mottel Ashkenazi, the head of the Raissin Talmudical Academy and Rabbi Avraham Osher Mostelin, the head of the Karlin Talmudical Academy. The four rooms, which were situated near the grave of Rabbi Meir Baal HaNess, were improved during the years 1878 and 1879, and additional rooms added. These improvements were made possible through the generosity of two benefactors, Reb Jonah Zeidav, who lived in Kiev, and his brother-in-law, Reb Avraham, who was from Berdichev. Contemporary records refer to the sterling work in the field of public health carried out at that time by the secretary of the charity group, Reb Avraham Beck. However, in spite of his devoted work, no solution was found to the ever-present problem of medical care in Tiberias at that time. In addition to the resident Jewish population of 2,500 people, hundreds of other Jews flocked to Tiberias in the hope that the hot springs would cure their ailments. In order to alleviate this problem, in 1881 the Jewish religious leaders of Tiberias published an appeal calling on benefactors outside Eretz Yisrael to contribute funds in order to establish a hospital in Tiberias. To this call were added the names of the Jewish religious leaders of Safed, Hebron and Jerusalem, and a number of doctors and the British consul in Jerusalem lent their support to the appeal.

Thus, in the year 1881, a new epoch in the history of medical care in Tiberias was begun, and this work expanded during the years 1883 and 1884. However, regrettably, a dispute arose among the leaders of the appeal. Reb Avraham Beck was of the opinion that they should not set their aims too high, and should be satisfied with improving the existing rooms that were already in use as a clinic, and that only one doctor and a pharmacist should be employed. On the other hand, Reb Shlomo Yosef Eliah maintained that they should aim for the establishment of a large and even luxurious hospital. This dispute is fully reported in the local press of the time.

As a result of this dispute, a Jewish hospital was not established in Tiberias at that time. Moreover, and even worse, a Scottish Christian missionary took advantage of the situation and in 1884 established a clinic with a resident doctor. Afterwards, this "missionary clinic" was enlarged and converted into a hospital. The situation of the Jews in Tiberias deteriorated greatly as a result of these developments. In 1886 a resident of Tiberias, Ephraim Neimark, wrote: "Other cities in our land have succeeded in finding generous benefactors who have been willing to finance the expenses required in order to employ doctors, but our communal leaders hold back, because they do not wish to reveal our troubles in public. Thus they leave the field open to the missionaries and their doctor. They have already purchased a large site for the construction of a hospital and a school. What will be the end of this no one can tell!"

A contemporary also described the work of the Mission. He stated that it began its work in 1879 and tried to win over the trust of the Jewish people in a cunning way. In its first year, the doctor employed by the mission merely requested payment for his treatment and for his advice, and never mentioned the work of the Mission. When, after a year of working in this manner, he had gained the confidence of his patients, he began to campaign also on behalf of the Mission. However, the writer was at pains to remind his readers that he was in no way criticising the poor Jews who visited the missionary clinic, as the missionary doctor was the only one in the town!

This situation continued for a number of years. In 1889, we read that the son of the energetic Reb Avraham Beck called on the leaders of the town of Tiberias to join together in order to bring to the town a well-qualified doctor "so as to remove the plague of the mission," since the mission doctor, "before he begins to cure the bodies of the sick Jewish patients, first tries to cure their souls." He adds that if the missionary doctor is away from the town for any reason, the poor patients are simply left to die, since they do not have enough money to travel to Safed where there is another doctor.

The situation only began to improve in 1890. In that year a writer in the local press reported that the leaders of the town had succeeded in engaging the services of a Jewish doctor, Dr. Hillel Jaffe, at a salary of 130 "napoleons" per annum (the local currency at the time). Later the same writer reported that the new doctor had restored the clinic, and that it was now ready to receive patients. He concluded that he hoped that "the benefactors among the children of Abraham our Father will feel the necessity of donating generously in order to help us to carry out this great religious deed."

Other appeals for funds written by leading citizens of Tiberias of that time were found to be preserved in the archives of University College, London, and were brought to Israel recently by the author Mr. Binyamin Kluger. Also at University College, London, were found two letters written by Chassidic leaders of the time, The Admor of Belz, Rabbi Yehoshua Rokeach, and the Admor of Sieniewa, Rabbi Yehezkel Shraga Halberstam. The letters, which were both written in German, called for donations for the hospital in Tiberias. The Admor from Belz wrote to a person unknown to us as follows:

Belz, 28 June 1892 (3rd Tammuz 5653)

I send you heartfelt greetings. I wish to write to you concerning the Rabbi bearing this letter, who is travelling far and wide in order to obtain contributions in order to establish a hospital in Tiberias in the Holy Land. Apart from the fact that we are strictly commanded in the Torah to help the sick, this particular case is exceptionally important, since we must liberate large numbers of our people from the influence of the Mission. The bearer of this letter will explain the situation to you verbally. Thus, in order to achieve this purpose, very heavy expenses are involved, and it would be a very great action if every person would at once give a generous donation so that the building of the hospital can proceed. Besides this, each person should promise an annual contribution. I myself have donated 50 florins to this cause.

With sincerest blessings to you, and may Jerusalem be rebuilt!

Yehoshua from Belz

A balance sheet of the fund's income and expenses was attached which recorded a contribution of 50 florins from the Admor of Belz.

The letter from the Admor of Sieniewa went as follows:

Sieniewa, 1st July 1892 (6th Tammuz 5653)

The Rabbi bearing this letter is working very hard in connection with the fulfilment of a very worthy aim as commanded by the Holy Torah — namely, the establishment of a hospital for the sick who visit the hot springs of Tiberias, and for the appointment of a qualified doctor in the town. This aim is all the more important, as Jewish people who visit the place in order to find a cure are obliged to visit the hospital established by missionaries. These missionaries employ doctors and distribute free medicines in order to entrap Jewish souls. Thus, as soon as a Jewish hospital is established, with doctors who will distribute medicines paid for by Jewish contributions, we will announce that it is forbidden for Jews to visit the hospital set up by the missionaries. Thus, every person is obligated to support this cause, each according to his ability.

In the hope of a perfect Redemption,

Yehezkel Shraga Halberstam

Attached to the two letters was a detailed balance sheet showing income and expenses for a complete year. Among the contributions listed are donations from residents of Munkatsch, Sotmer, Heidelberg, Budapest, Amsterdam, London, Liverpool, Antwerp and Paris, and it is recorded that the Rav from Brisk, resident in Jerusalem, donated 25 francs. In the list of expenses is mentioned the annual salary of Dr. Hillel Jaffe, postal and office expenses, and contributions given to the poor and sick of Tiberias.

The following note is appended at the bottom of the balance sheet:

We wish to inform you that Dr. Hillel Jaffe is leaving Tiberias, and we are making great efforts in order to find another Jewish doctor to replace him. We have sent out letters and appeals to every quarter to find a doctor who will be willing to come here. It is indeed most upsetting to report that until now we have not succeeded in finding another doctor. We seek a Jewish doctor, fully qualified, with all the diplomas required by the Turkish authorities.

The annual salary offered is between 100 and 150 napoleons. Extra payment will be made for home visits.

The news of the intention of Dr. Hillel Jaffe to leave Tiberias brought much sorrow and concern to the Jews of Tiberias. Dr. Jaffe (the modern Hillel Jaffe Hospital and Medical Centre in Hadera, Israel, is named after him), faithfully treated the sick of Tiberias for two years, and won universal approval and high praise for his devotion and skill. Once again the Jewish leaders of Tiberias sent out appeals to contributors living outside Eretz Yisrael, advising them of the plight of the sick of Tiberias and of the dangers of the activities of the Mission.

In 1894, the leaders of Tiberias succeeded in finding a replacement for Dr. Jaffe in the person of Dr. Rothstein, and in 1895 a second doctor, Dr. Shimon Muell, was also appointed.

The appointment of these two doctors did much to improve the condition of the sick of Tiberias. However, it did not provide a complete solution to the problems created by the fact that a population which had now grown to 3,000 persons did not have a hospital within reach. In 1895, it was rumoured that Baron Rothschild had appreciated the great need and had promised to construct a large hospital in Tiberias, in the hope that other benefactors would help him in financing this project. However, it appeared that this rumour was not based on fact. Help came, in fact, from an unforeseen quarter. The local paper in Tiberias at that time carried the following announcement: "After all the bitter conflicts through which we have passed in our town, how happy we are to announce the following good news. Mr. Yehoshua Usvosky, the chief civil servant in charge of the Rosh Pina and Galilee settlements, has brought peace to our town. He has succeeded in constructing some beautiful dwellings which are clean and well ventilated, with modern open windows, the cost of which is being financed from a fund donated by that princely benefactor, Reb Haim Eliezer Poliakov (a wealthy banker and industrialist who was the President of the Jewish community of Moscow at that time) and his charming wife, Madame Raissa Poliakov. The finance is now fully available for this magnificent project. This will be an outstanding symbol of the benefactor's kindness to the poor and sick of our holy town, and also to the sick of Jerusalem, Safed and Hebron, both those living in the old settlements and those coming from the new settlements, and indeed to the sick from all over the world who come to bathe in the hot springs of Tiberias, and who find in them a remedy for their illnesses and a comfort for their troubled souls. Thus our honoured Mr. Usvosky was the person who was privileged to fulfil this lofty aim for which we have longed for for so many years, and in addition he has succeeded in bringing to Tiberias a highly qualified doctor, Dr. Moshe Goldberg.

However, to our great sorrow, we are once again faced with the problem of how to meet the gigantic expenses which will now be involved in the running of the new hospital. Thus, once again we have to turn to the generous benefactors among the children of Abraham our Father to send us their contributions for the support of this holy project."

The Hospital Founded by Rabbi Akiva Eger

Meyer Wunder

Summary: When the Grand Rabbi of Sanz, *ztz"l*, founded the Laniado Hospital in Netanya, he was following a Jewish historical tradition whereby great Torah leaders and Rabbis establish hospitals which they administer strictly in accordance with the rulings of the Torah. Meyer Wunder relates the history of another such institution founded by Rabbi Akiva Eger in Posen in the year 1830. The hospital, which never departed from the Torah-true regulations laid down by Rabbi Akiva Eger, flourished and expanded right up to the destruction of the Jewish community there by the Germans in the Holocaust.

Biographical note: Rabbi Akiva Eger, whose scholarly Rabbinical works are still studied and quoted by rabbinical and talmudical students throughout the world, was born in Hungary in the year 1761. In 1816 he was elected to be the Rabbi of Posen, where he served until his death in 1838. He is recognised as being one of the greatest of Jewish teachers and Rabbis. At his request, the following words were recorded on his gravestone: "Here lies our Rabbi, Rabbi Akiva Eger, who served those who were servants of Hashem."

The years during which Rabbi Akiva Eiger served as the Rabbi of Posen were filled with study of the Torah, and with the performance of good deeds. Hundreds of eager students flocked to learn Torah from him, and many of them later became Rabbis and Judges in Jewish communities throughout the world. His Talmudical College was too small to take in all who wished to learn there. In addition, there existed no

Jewish hospital in the area. In the year 1830, the solution to these two problems was found through the generosity of Reb Shlomo Binyamin Latz, one of the leading members of the Jewish community of Posen at that time, and a devoted follower of Rabbi Akiva Eger. He was taken ill and felt that his end was approaching. He asked Rabbi Akiva Eiger to visit him, and told him that he intended to leave a large sum of money which should be devoted to the building of a hospital and a Talmudical College. He appointed Rabbi Akiva Eiger to be executor of his estate, and instructed him to use two-thirds of the money left for the building of the hospital, and one third for the building of the Talmudical College. It was stated in his will that the administration of the hospital should be under the sole direction and supervision of Rabbi Akiva Eger, and a clause in the will emphasised that the secular leaders of the Jewish community should have no influence on the running of the hospital. The sick man stated in his will: "I have complete trust in the saintliness, great Torah learning and perfect honesty of Rabbi Akiva Eiger, and I request that all his wishes should be followed as if they were my own."

Rabbi Akiva Eger purchased a two-storey building from the money left in the will. The building was called "The House of Shlomo," after the first name of the donor. One wing of the building, comprising thirteen rooms, was devoted for use as the hospital, and the remaining rooms made up the Talmudical College. Rabbi Akiva Eger supervised every detail of the construction of the hospital and laid down detailed regulations as to how it should be administered. Hundreds of sick people from all the neighbouring areas were treated in the hospital. Each of the sick were asked to pay only a very small fee, and the poor were given free treatment.

Nevertheless, the hospital finances were never in deficit,

since Rabbi Akiva Eger obtained large donations from generous Jewish people, and they never had to ask for financial assistance from the secular leaders of the Jewish community. This displeased the secular leaders, who were already strongly influenced by "modern" anti-traditional and "Reform" views. They sent a letter of complaint to the government of the country in which they claimed that the hospital was in a state of neglect, that its administration was not being carried out efficiently, and that Rabbi Akiva Eger was taking hospital funds and using them for his personal needs. They maintained that the law of the land stated that all Jewish communal institutions had to be under the sole control of the secular communal leaders. They therefore requested that Rabbi Akiva Eger should be removed from his position as head of the institutions, and that they should be transferred into their control.

Rabbi Akiva Eger sent the government a long reply to these accusations, in which he related how the hospital and Talmudical College had been founded, and claimed that he administered the institutions correctly in accordance with the law of the land. He added: "I forgive those who attack me with my whole heart, but I am deeply upset that they gave into their weaknesses in this matter." The government authorities asked if they could examine the written regulations on which the hospital administration was based, and also sent an expert to carry out a full inspection of the hospital. The government inspector afterwards stated in his report: "I found this institution to be in outstandingly good order. The sick people are very pleased with the treatment they receive. I found everything correctly set out in the best possible taste in every part of the building. The secular leaders of the community should be rebuked for the attitude they have taken."

The secular leaders tried to persuade the government to

decree that after Rabbi Akiva Eger had passed away, the administration of the hospital should be changed and placed in their control. Rabbi Akiva Eger bitterly attacked this suggestion. He quoted the seven or eight regulations upon which the administration of the hospital was based, and stated: "I want to be absolutely sure that at all times in the future the administration of the hospital will be based upon these regulations. I strongly hope that the government will understand and support my wishes."

The hospital Rabbi Akiva Eger had founded flourished for many years. It was replaced later by a large modern hospital built from funds donated by another member of the community.

However, the original building remained, and was converted into a home for the aged. In fact, the administration of the hospital did pass into the hands of "Reform" Jews, but, to everyone's surprise, they did not change a single one of the regulations laid down by Rabbi Akiva Eger for the administration of the institution. The hospital actually retained its complete independence right up to the time of the destruction of the community by the Germans in the Holocaust. An historian of the period has recorded the words that were engraved on the marble stone set up over the entrance to the hospital. They were: " 'The House of Shlomo' founded by the outstanding philanthropist, the late Shlomo Zalman Binyamin Latz, in the year 1830. Our great revered teacher and Rabbi Akiva Eger, established and set up everything here in his great wisdom in the year 1834. May their memories be for a blessing and may their righteousness live forever!"